Did you know...?

The **ADHD Awareness Book Project** is an ongoing effort to bring the best tips and strategies, and now also stories, from the world's top ADHD experts, to you in an easily digestible format. The series includes:

- *365 Ways to Succeed with ADHD (2011)*
- *365+1 Ways to Succeed with ADHD (2012)*
- *More Ways to Succeed with ADHD (2013)*
- *Inspirational Ways to Succeed with ADHD (2014)*
- *Wacky Ways to Succeed with ADHD (2015)*

Each book contains unique content and follows a "bite-sized" format for easy reading. By adding all **five Amazon #1 Bestselling** books to your collection, you will have over 1000 unique ADHD strategies and stories at your fingertips! With such a large variety, you are guaranteed to discover a number of tips and/or stories that will make the difference!

This series is the <u>perfect gift</u> for yourself, a loved, or an ADHD professional you know.

Order all five editions at www.CoachingforADHD.com

Praise for the ADHD Awareness Book Project!

"Whether you have ADHD or are supporting someone with ADHD there is something for everyone in The ADHD Awareness Book Project. This series is an excellent resource! There has been a need for this type of book for a long time. Now, it is finally here!!!"

> ~**David Giwerc,** Founder & President, ADD Coach Academy, author of Permission to Proceed: The Keys to Creating a Life of Passion, Purpose and Possibility for Adults with ADHD

"Full of wit and wisdom! Brilliant best tips from some of the best in the field and short enough to be read and appreciated by even those with ADHD who hate to read. Love it!

> ~**Michelle Novotni,** Ph.D. ADHD Expert; Psychologist and ADHD coach and author of What Do Other People Know that I Don't

"I meet all kinds of people with a creeping sense that their attention is out of whack. Laurie's books are perfect for a daily dose of awareness for the diagnosed ADDer, the self-diagnosed, and those who are ADDish or chronically disorganized. You'll love them for both practicality and humor."

> ~ **Judith Kolberg**, Author, Conquering Chronic Disorganization and ADD-Friendly Ways to Organize Your Life, www.squallpress.net

"Read 365+1 ways to succeed with ADHD, and Laurie's other books, and you'll quickly develop an interesting, new ADHD recovery vocabulary. 'Comprehensive' is one new and essential ADHD evaluation and treatment word. ADHD, as you know, is more complex than a simple set of labels, and treatment/recovery requires a careful review of multiple

issues, many covered in the deeply comprehensive pages of Laurie's books. From my perspective, 365+1 Ways to Succeed with ADHD is the singular most comprehensive ADHD recovery book available, and I strongly encourage you to read and listen to the abundant array of national experts who provided their best insights for your next recovery steps."

~ **Dr. Charles Parker**, Psychiatrist and Psycho pharmacologist at Core Psych and Author of New ADHD Medication Rules

"Laurie Dupar has done it again with this new amazing compilation of wisdom from the top experts and practitioners in the field. Just like her first book, this new one is infused with her positive view. Laurie Dupar's devotion to helping people with ADHD live rewarding and strength-based lives is evident. I have her first book in my waiting room, and I frequently see clients pick it up for a few minutes before their appointments, turn randomly to a new page, and always find something that speaks just to them. This new book delivers equally practical wisdom in bite-size pieces. A reader will always find something to help them at the right time in an extremely ADHD friendly format."

~ **Sari Solden**, Psychotherapist, MS, LMFT, and Author of Women with Attention Deficit Disorder and Journeys Through ADD

With much appreciation and respect to my core team members, Meg Gehan and Shaun Roney!

Your support, resourcefulness and sense of humor make these books possible!

Thank you from the bottom of my heart!

~ Laurie Dupar

The ADHD Awareness Book

Project

WACKY Ways to

Succeed with ADHD

THE NEVER BEFORE TOLD FUN, OUT-OF-THE-BOX SECRETS THAT WILL GET YOU SMILING AND SURVIVING WITH ADHD

Laurie Dupar, PMHMP, RN, PCC

Wacky Ways to Succeed with ADHD

Publisher: Laurie Dupar, Herding Cats Press

Granite Bay, CA

Cover Design by Jodi Burgess Design

Content editing by Linda Barnett-Johnson,
writingfriend@yahoo.com

About The ADHD Awareness Book Project

"Never doubt that a small group of thoughtful, committed, people can change the world. Indeed it is the only thing that ever has."

~Margaret Mead

The ADHD Awareness Book Project began five years ago with these goals: provide people with ADHD valuable strategies and tips to help them succeed, and increase the awareness of ADHD world-wide, all in an ADHD-friendly format!

We have come a long way in our understanding of ADHD, considering that in 1902 symptoms consistent with ADHD were labeled a "morbid defect of moral control"! We have come to understand that ADHD is neither gender nor ethnic specific and is not something individuals out-grow. However, the fact that ADHD is a real and lifelong disorder has not yet made enough of an impact on the overall awareness or successful daily management of ADHD symptoms and challenges.

Too often I hear from people all over the world—parents, students and newly diagnosed adults—who are struggling alone, not knowing that answers to their challenges are available. Many have never heard the term 'ADHD' and they have no idea that by learning to do things in ways that better fit their ADHD brain-style, they could succeed . . . at just about anything!

After 13 years of specializing in ADHD, and over 25 years working in mental health, the continued lack of awareness about ADHD, and the limited availability of resources, is no longer acceptable to me. Frankly, I am tired. I am tired of knowing that individuals, from young children to adults in their 70s, are struggling alone with ADHD, unaware that there are answers, resources, hope and help out here. I have decided to be part of the solution by publishing these books, and I am not alone.

Nearly five years ago, believing in the power of community and the dedication of my colleagues in the ADHD community, I announced that I would be coordinating a book of tips and strategies for succeeding with ADHD, featuring as many ADHD experts as possible. I invited all the ADHD professionals I knew, and asked them to invite ADHD professionals they knew, to participate in this project. In the first *ADHD Awareness Book Project,* titled *365 Ways to Succeed with ADHD*, over 80 co-authors from a variety of professions responded to my request and submitted their answers to the question: "What is the best tip or strategy you have to help someone with ADHD succeed?"

In its second edition, titled *365+1 Ways to Succeed with ADHD,* the *ADHD Awareness Book Project* expanded to incorporate contributing experts from all over the globe, including South Africa, Turkey, Sweden, Denmark and Ireland. Our experts included 'junior experts', like eight-year-olds, and 'senior experts', like 78-year-olds, sharing valuable tips and strategies to help people with ADHD succeed.

In its third edition, *MORE Ways to Succeed with ADHD,* we answered the call again for "more". More unique ways, tips, strategies and ideas to help better manage ADHD.

In this fourth edition, *Inspirational Ways to Succeed with ADHD,* alongside the brand-new tips and strategies, we have added powerful, uplifting stories about ADHD from people just like you.

And now, our fifth edition appreciates the creative side of persons living with ADHD, focusing on out-of-the-box strategies and wacky, fun ways people with ADHD compensate for their ADHD challenges. I know that within these pages you will find the one specific tip, strategy or story that will be the answer you are most needing in this moment.

How <u>YOU</u> are making a difference when you buy this book!

Whether this book is for you or for someone you care about, a portion of the sales of *The ADHD Awareness Book Project: Inspirational Ways to Succeed with ADHD* will be used to support three international ADHD organizations:

- Children and Adults with Attention Deficit/Hyperactivity Disorder (CHADD)
- Attention Deficit Disorder Association (ADDA)
- ADHD Coaches Organization (ACO)

Thank you for purchasing this book, being part of the solution, and helping us to increase awareness of ADHD!

~ *Laurie Dupar*

Contact the Contributors

As you read through these pages and find particular strategies useful, or stories inspiring, I encourage you to connect with the contributors. They look forward to hearing from you!

How to Use this Book

Our books are intended to be 'ADHD friendly.' They are formatted to include a large variety of tips and stories that are short, succinct, easy to read and immediately useable.

Some of you may want to put this book by your bedside and read one tip a day . . . Terrific! Some of you may sit down and read the entire book in one sitting . . . Have fun! Still others, in your very wonderful ADHD style, may thumb through the book, starting wherever it catches your attention, reading from the middle to the end . . . , the end to the middle . . . , or even every other page! It is yours to decide. Enjoy this book in whatever manner your wonderful ADHD brain chooses!

Contents

About The ADHD Awareness Book Project ....*i*

How to Use this Book ....*v*

Dedication ....*xvii*

Acknowledgements ....*xix*

Introduction ....*xxi*

Loving and Creating a Perfect Storm
Holly Metzger *3*

Changing it Up – Recognizing What Works
Sherri Dettmer Cannon *4*

Doing the Lesser of Two Awfuls ... *Laurie Dupar* *7*

It's Only an Experiment!
Elizabeth Ahmann *8*

Use the Cloud
Valerie C. Krupp *9*

Get a Coach   *Laurie Dupar* *10*

Motivate with the ADHD Trifecta   *Casey Dixon* *11*

Organization Makes the Grade
Cheryl Feuer Gedzelman. *13*

The Ultimate Parent's Question
Diane Dempster & Elaine Taylor-Klaus *15*

Planned Procrastination   *Laurie Dupar* *16*

The Biggest Difference?   *Roxanne Fouché* *17*

For Your ADHD, Apologize Not! *Jeremy Didier* 20

Red is the Color of My Heart *Laurie Dupar* 23

Buzz Ya Later: Tools To Tame Your Time Optimism
Kate Barrett...24

Finding the Upside to Keep From Getting Down *Dr. Billi*...25

Follow That Squirrel! *Judy A. MacNamee*...........................27

How to Find an ADHD Coach *Laurie Dupar*......................28

How Working in a Noisy Place Actually Works!
Carlene Bauwens 29

The Focus Formula *Michele Toner*.......................................33

ADHD Writing!?! Wacky Happy WACKY ADHD
Michael Alan Schuler 34

Get There on Time *Laurie Dupar* 37

Skyping Through the House We Go! *Candace Sahm*...........38

Communicate Wisely - With Wacky Words!?
Melissa R. Farhney 39

The Toilet Paper Test
Diane Dempster & Elaine Taylor-Klaus 40

ADHD and Entrepreneurs *Laurie Dupar*............................41

Just One Meaningful Word *Angelis Iglesias* 42

ADHD ~ It Can Happen to Anybody! *Roya Kravetz*..........43

Smile to Focus *Ariel Davis* 46

Lazy Susan Homework *Laurie Dupar* 48

That's it!!! Get to Your Room and Get a Game –
I'll Be in There in 2 Minutes with a Snack!
Cindy Goldrich... 49

Fifty Shades of Grey *Michele Toner* 50

A Wacky Way to Think Clearly *Alan Brown* 53

Found It! It's In My Pants! *Kari Miller* 55

Considering Becoming an ADHD Coach?
Laurie Dupar.. 56

The LEGO Meltdown
Jennifer E. Kampfe 57

Birds of a Feather *Roxanne Fouché* 60

Counting Goals in Days *Laurie Dupar* 62

Spinning Top Spinning Colors
Michael Alan Schuler 63

ADHD Hometown Heroines *Kari Miller* 68

Kitchens are for Brushing Teeth! *Jeremy Didier* 71

When You Love Someone with ADHD *Laurie Dupar* 72

ADHD Color Blind Celebrating
Michael Alan Schuler 74

Hypnotize Yourself to Peace of Mind!
Anna Marie Lindell 76

Jump Start Motivation *Roxanne Fouché*...........................77

Stop Feeling Guilty and Take a Nap *Carlene Bauwens* 78

Popsicle Stick Chores *Laurie Dupar* *80*

Stop Interruptions & Teach Patient Waiting
Diane Dempster & Elaine Taylor-Klaus *81*

Changing the Game Plan – Becoming Good Enough
Billi Bittan *82*

The Secret of Connection *Jared & DeAnn Jennette* *84*

Let Freedom Ring, Not the Phone! *Laurie Dupar* *85*

The Duplicated (ADHD) Life *Linda Roggli* *87*

Making Space for Original Thinking
Sherri Dettmer Cannon *88*

Did Curiosity Kill Kat...or Give New Life?
Katie Blum-Katz *89*

What's Your "Study Style?" *Laurie Dupar* *91*

Red Nose Day *Barb Rosenfeld* *93*

Self-Efficacy For All Women *Kari Miller* *94*

Special Spot (Keeping Safe)   *Pat Corbett* *97*

Solving Hour-Long Showers *Laurie Dupar* *98*

Need a Vacation? *Elizabeth Ahmann* *100*

Wiggle While You Work *Scott Ertl* *101*

When the Floor is the Biggest Shelf in the Room
Laurie Dupar *102*

Don't Feed the Trolls *Michele Toner* 103

The 3 WACKIEST Things About Having ADHD
Roya Kravetz 106

Avoiding Something? *Elizabeth Ahmann* 107

My "Brains" *Laurie Dupar* 108

Calming the Senses *Pat Corbett* 109

The Power of Empathy *Jared & DeAnn Jennette* 111

Stories Brought Me Up *Angelis Iglesias* 112

What is Your Rainbow Play List? *Laurie Dupar* 115

Handling Stress: Mine! *Pat Corbett*................................116

Five Communication Secrets That Can Change Your ADHD
Relationship Forever *Linda Roggli*...................................118

Surprise! Wake Up Brain! *Kari Miller* 120

Beat the Blues *Laurie Dupar*..121

Make a Micro-Change *Casey Dixon* 122

Find Your Zen Where You Can *Anne Marie Nantais*........125

Why Did I Come Into This Room? *Silvia Razon*.................128

Time Outs are Not Just for Toddlers *Laurie Dupar* 129

Desktop Dopamine Dosers *Kari Miller* 130

Don't Hit Yourself on the Way Down! *Sarah D. Wright*..132

Put on Your War Glitter *Laurie Dupar* 133

The Shadow Game *Pat Corbett*..134

Do You Want to Be Right or Happy?
Diane Dempster & Elaine Taylor-Klaus..............................135

The Monster Binder *Cheryl Feuer Gedzelman*.................. 137

Are You Jet Lagged? *Laurie Dupar*....................................140

I Know I Put it Someplace! *Steven Freedman*...................141

Don't Worry, Your Child Will Get Distracted. Or You Will.
Jared & DeAnn Jennette..142

Create an Action Board! *Laurie Dupar*.............................144

Forget Me Not
Stephanie J. Noel Kirlin...145

ADHD and Rockin' It! *Candace Sahm*...............................146

Making a Focus Bubble *Pat Corbett*..................................147

Is Your "Filter" Full? *Laurie Dupar*..................................148

Your Seven (Yes Seven!) Senses *Ariel Davis*......................149

Please Don't Make Me Adult *Sanlia Marais*.......................151

Pause to Ponder Positively *Laurie Dupar*.........................153

Mind Mapping in Reverse *Valerie C. Krupp*................... 155

Don't Teach Kids to Lie (or How to Teach Kids NOT to Lie)
Diane Dempster & Elaine Taylor-Klaus.............................156

Keeping Focused (Textbooks) *Pat Corbett*.........................157

Scribbles, Scrawls and Solutions (to Truly Horrible
Handwriting) *Linda Roggli*...158

An ADHD Conundrum *Laurie Dupar* 159

From Our Family to Yours *Pat Corbett* 160

Tom Sawyer Knew a Thing or Two *Sarah D. Wright* 161

Just Laugh!...It Could Be Worse *Karen A. Timm*..............162

Neurodiversity: It's How You Frame It! *Cindy Goldrich* .163

Coffee Pot Alarm Clocks *Laurie Dupar*........................... 164

ADHD & Lost Jewelry *Judi Jerome*...................................165

You Yelled - Get to the Jar! *Cindy Goldrich* 169

My Career with ADHD- A Simple Love Story
Shell Mendelson 170

Did You Wake Up on the "Bad Side" of the Brain?
Laurie Dupar..174

??ADHD or ADHD or ADHDDH!!
Michael Alan Schuler 175

Sanity Restored *Veronica Taylor*...................................... 181

Don't Forget the Fun! *Jared & DeAnn Jennette* 182

Time to Play (Everyday)! *Elizabeth Ahmann* 183

Whine Your Way to a Happy Career With ADHD
Shell Mendelson 184

Sing and Dance Your Way Through Any Task
Valerie C. Krupp 186

First: Attention - Then: Directions *Pat Corbett* 187

Bright Shiny Coach Syndrome ©   *Laurie Dupar* 188

A Spoonful of Sugar *Angelis Iglesias*...................189

What, Me Study? *Ariel Davis* 190

Are You a Helicopter Partner? *Laurie Dupar* 193

Lock Away Success *Stephanie J. Noel Kirlin*....................194

What's Emoji Got to do With It? *Candace Sahm* 195

Be Imperfect on Purpose *Margit Crane Luria*.................197

Hidden Highlights *Laurie Dupar*.........................198

ADD Yin Yang *Zion Banks* 199

Just Breathe: Self-Regulation for Parents
Jared & DeAnn Jennette...................................200

Mindfulness for ADHD? No Way? *Casey Dixon*...............201

Do You Brush Your Teeth? *Laurie Dupar* 203

Tag! I'm It! *Billi Bittan* 204

The Day the Frogs Flew *Michele Toner*...........................205

Finding Fun *Pat Corbett* 208

Do You Suffer From Time Zone Dyscalculia?
Laurie Dupar... 209

Tipping into Technology *Stephanie J. Noel Kirlin*............210

What Do You Mean, Focus??? *Elizabeth Ahmann* 211

Sticker Art Motivation Tip *Kari Miller*.............................212

Extra Exploration Time   *Pat Corbett*..................................*213*

Are You Time Blind? *Laurie Dupar* *214*

Dedication

This book is dedicated to people living with ADHD, wherever you are. Your commitment, perseverance and determination to find answers about how to live successfully with ADHD are a constant source of inspiration. YOU are the experts. YOU are the source for what we know "works" and what, even though it might make sense, doesn't.

This book is also dedicated to ADHD professionals who are committed to making a positive difference in the lives of people with ADHD. These experts include: doctors, therapists, nutritionists and dieticians, coaches, educators, lawyers, accountants, organizational specialists and many more. Many of you chose to share your expertise by contributing to this book. Thank you all. I am proud to be your colleague.

Individually, we make a difference in the lives of people with ADHD. Together, there is limitless possibility to positively change the world's understanding and awareness of ADHD. This book could not have happened without ALL of you. Thank you.

Acknowledgements

Putting this book together was a labor of love, borne by a passion to make a positive difference in the lives of people with ADHD. In fact, I can say it has been with an 'ADHD spirit' that for the past five years, the books of *The ADHD Awareness Book Project* have been written and published. Five years ago I had an idea, and I was determined to make it a reality without thought to any obstacles, roadblocks, nay-sayers or disbelievers. Fore-most in my thoughts has always been you, the people I both have met and have yet to meet who live with ADHD.

With you always on my mind, I was determined to do what someone with ADHD would do: find a way through the obstacles, keep an eye on the goal despite its seeming impossibility, and get up each day determined and hopeful to succeed. You are the inspiration. Thank you.

I also want to thank all of the contributors of *The ADHD Awareness Book Project: Wacky Ways to Succeed with ADHD*. Your individual and collective beliefs, support and contributions to this book have made it a reality. I am humbled by your commitment. And, of course, I want to thank my family, you know who you are. Without your constant belief in me, and your un-dying patience, this effort would not have been possible. I love you all. I also want to thank my assistant extraordinaire, Meg Gehan, who always has my back; Shaun Roney, who is a master at managing my media; Jodi Burgess at Jodi Burgess Design, who created the book cover; and Linda Barnett-Johnson at writingfriend@yahoo.com, whose expertise and craft with words helped all of our entries 'sparkle.' This wouldn't have been possible without each and all of you. Thank you!

~Laurie Dupar

Introduction

Fifteen years ago, my youngest son was diagnosed with ADHD. As a mental health professional used to having the answers, I uncharacteristically found myself searching for anything that would help me better understand this mental health disorder so that I could help him minimize his challenges and maximize his talents. At the time, resources were scarce. Several years later, I discovered ADHD coaching and saw how much of a difference this approach made in helping both of us reduce the struggles and, instead, experience success. Surprising even myself, becoming an ADHD coach and working with people having unique brain styles as they tap into their brilliance, has been my passion for the past 13 years. And my son? He is proudly completing five years of service in the United States Navy and looking forward to discovering the next chapter of his life, which will no doubt include his passions for fitness, adventure and travel.

I never set out to be an ADHD coach. Having earned my master's degree as a psychiatric mental health nurse practitioner, I was prepared to diagnose and treat the whole array of mental health disorders. I would have never believed that understanding, advocating or working with people diagnosed with ADHD would have been so all-consuming and rewarding. Yet, I have been amazed with the consistent and never-slowing stream of people challenged with this disorder. As an ADHD coach, I get to work with some of the most amazingly brilliant and creative people every day . . . and these are just my clients. The experts, professionals and specialists who focus on working with people diagnosed with ADHD are equally as incredible.

ADHD is a 24/7 disorder impacting the ability of affected individuals to focus, pay attention, plan, prioritize ... and a whole host of other challenges. For some people with ADHD, it is difficult to complete less interesting tasks like homework, bills, organizing or planning. The inability to complete these tasks often creates huge disorder and chaos in their lives. For others, throughout the day, from the moment of waking to the hours of trying to fall asleep, daily life can be a struggle, whether to find motivation or to fight distractions due to an inner sense of restlessness. That's the thing about ADHD.... It is so different for everyone.

A number of amazing international organizations are available to help people better understand ADHD. I am proud that a portion of the proceeds of the book sales of *The ADHD Awareness Book Project* goes to support these organizations. I encourage you to seek out the resources of such organizations as Children and Adults with Attention

Deficit Disorder (CHADD), www.chadd.org; Adults with Attention Deficit Disorder Association (ADDA), www.add.org; and the ADHD Coaches Organization (ACO), www.adhdcoaches.org

In addition, many books are available by authors who really understand the challenges of ADHD, some of whom have contributed to this book. I encourage you to explore their wisdom. I believe we can never know too much about ADHD.

And last, but not least, there are individual professionals who serve the ADHD community. Coaches, doctors, researchers, therapists, nutritionists, educators, lawyers, and others. Over the years, I have been awed at this community's dedication and commitment to serve, each individual, each using unique strengths, talents and gifts, in his or her own way, to improve the lives of people with ADHD.

Wacky Ways to Succeed with ADHD is our fifth book. The first book, *365 Ways to Succeed with ADHD*, the second, *365+1 Ways to Succeed with ADHD* and the third, *MORE ways to Succeed with ADHD,* and the fourth, *Inspirational Ways to Succeed with ADHD* each achieved a #1 ranking in their category on Amazon.com. We hope this will be a #1 resource for you as well!

The ADHD Awareness Book Project has been an opportunity for many experts to come together in one place to share their 'gems' with you. It is written with parents, families, children, teachers, teens, college students and adults of all ages in mind. There is literally something for everyone!

Drawing from their wide varieties of expertise and experience, contributing experts have offered you their best out-of-the-box strategies and tips to help you succeed with ADHD. I know you will enjoy and find value in all of their contributions.

*"I will keep telling you
that you are important, deserving,
loving, intelligent, worthy,
compassionate, beautiful, creative,
inspiring, brave, true, strong, and
able until you finally
realize it for yourself."*

~Anonymous

Loving and Creating
a Perfect Storm

To create the perfect storm, it takes the necessary ingredients, just like it takes the right formula for the ADHD mind to get hyper-focused. Storms can last a short or long amount of time and can be very unpredictable; however, there is one thing that is always consistent: they come to an end. To be the most productive, it's very crucial to love and take advantage of moments when you get into the zone. How do you accomplish tasks if there is limited internal push to complete them? I have developed a few tricks to create storms to generate motivation and get focused.

1. Place sticky notes on my desk with things I need to complete
2. Look at my binder of accomplishments and successful projects
3. Set a timer to do something for ten minutes
4. Create imaginary deadlines
5. Develop a routine block schedule

~ Holly Metzger, M.Ed., CSA

Holly Metzger is a Youth Fitness Director, Tennis Coach and Certified Tennis Instructor who specializes in developing and instructing youth fitness and sports programs. www.hctennis.com

Changing it Up – Recognizing What Works

Like a lot of us with ADHD, I used to keep my wackiness on internal lock-down, wanting my brain to work like those of the neurotypicals around me. Instead, I got indigestion and I couldn't find my creative self at all. Here's what I know now:

1. I Fling my Bits. Most of the time, a jaunty conga line of half-thoughts gyrates across my brain. These waft about and play hard to get. Then I hired Jennifer, who studied my ways and said, "Fling your bits to me. They're great bits. I'll sort them." Now, I email these bits, trusting my "receiver" to catch them and help me tame the idea tsunami. My projects are now more reflective of me, and of course more fun.

2. Physicians' Waiting Rooms Inspire Me. I used to chase my brain hoping to trick it into working with me. Then I noticed when and where my richest insights emerged. My list included blow-drying hair, walking, and sitting in medical waiting rooms. So I built these in – arriving 30 minutes early to write in my dentist's waiting area. I'm also fond of a spacious, outdoor parking lot where I park, open all the windows for the ocean breeze to blow, and alternate between writing and cleaning every corner of the car interior. It works like a charm. Wacky.

3. I'm Bringing My Stuff – All of It. My business requires frequent travel. For years, I've studied the relationship between how much stuff I bring and my happiness. When I pack small, I have only half the fun. I simply do not know today what I will feel like wearing tomorrow. It's also my past time to make the hotel room into a sacred, cozy space. This takes props. Recently, a room service waiter looked about and asked why I had twinkly white lights all over? "They make me happy and help me write," I said. He smiled and said, "Ah, I see – you are a writer."

4. Storm Cellar – Tornado Watch or Whatever It Takes. When she goes into research mode, Brené Brown sends family packing and "goes all Jackson Pollack." Me too. I hole up, and make an enormously big deal of the fact that I. Am. Not. Available. Nothing is to be expected of me during this time. As I construct this creative "bunker," the dopamine flows. I say goodbye to husband and cats, prepare the reward snacks, tape my plan to the wall, darken the room, string white lights, sit on the floor and break out fresh markers and play dough. Of note, when I used to act like my daunting project was no big deal, it grew into a VERY big, hairy deal. Now I deem it large and worthy of disrupting status quo from the start.

5. I Rely on my Tribe – Facilitating adult learning is the most fun I have. I'm in my zone, learning and laughing with my

group, fully present. When it came to the behind-the-scenes work of designing my own workshops however, I felt out of my league. Sitting at my desk alone and quiet (because that's how I imagined "others" did it), I tried to design a workshop. Not even twinkling white lights helped. Now, I meet my friend Terri in the bustling lobby of one particularly classy L.A. hotel. There, cross-legged on the floor, we brainstorm ideas and spend the day moving neon post-its about on the high glass wall overlooking poolside sunbathers. Turns out I'm good at this – as long as I honor my wacky truth: with a partner, out loud, hands-on and moving about.

~ Sherri Dettmer Cannon

Sherri Cannon, Executive Coach, ADHD Coach and seasoned workshop leader, has helped individuals and teams around the world thrive by leveraging strengths, collaboration and innovation since 1990. Diagnosed with ADHD in 2001, Sherri specializes in working with multi-function teams, business leaders and innovators of all kinds. In 2015, Sherri co-chaired ADHD Coaches Organization's 8th International Conference. As Master Facilitator of Fierce Conversations™ as well as certified StandOut -Strengths™ Facilitator and Coach, Sherri helps professionals leverage their unique strengths and build teams high in trust, innovation, fun and results. For more information, visit www.sherricannon.com

Doing the Lesser of Two Awfuls

Have you ever had those items on your to-do list that never get done? You know, the ones that feel overwhelming, boring or just plain yucky? If you are like me, these items are consistently being transferred to be done the next day, with little progress being made on completing them at all. Next time, try this trick!

When I have several items on my list and I am finding it difficult to get motivated. I focus on two of those challenging tasks. This eliminates the possibility of having something on my list that will distract me from getting those less attractive tasks done. Limiting my choices to these two items inevitably ends in at least one or both getting completed...or at the very least, an even lesser task, like cleaning my house gets accomplished in the process!

~Laurie Dupar, PMHNP, RN, PCC

Laurie Dupar, PMHNP, RN, PCC is a trained Psychiatric Nurse Practitioner and 12 year veteran ADHD coach specializing in mentoring and training emerging ADHD Coaches.
www.coachingforadhd.com support@coachingforadhd.com

It's Only an Experiment!

Often it's hard to try something new - even a potentially helpful strategy - because of fear of failure. This is understandable if you've experienced your share of failure in the past. At the same time, without trying anything new, you'll never find what works!

In these circumstances, I like to think about Thomas Edison. Although best known for inventing the light bulb, he experienced numerous failed experiments before finding success. His enlightening view was: "I have not failed. I've just found 10,000 ways that won't work."

With Edison in mind, re-framing new experiences as "experiments" can take some pressure off. Perhaps a new strategy will work! More likely, some parts of a strategy will work, but others will need to be tweaked. Still, if after trying, a strategy isn't a good fit, you've probably learned something. Then, like Edison, you can just head back to the drawing board.

~ Elizabeth (Liz) Ahmann, ScD, RN, ACC

Liz Ahmann, ScD, RN, ACC incorporates positive psychology into coaching with her clients and teaches mindfulness classes for individuals with ADHD. See: www.lizahmann.com ww.lizahmann.com/mindfulness.html

Use the Cloud

Stacks of paper are a BIG problem for ADDers. Bills, letters and other snail mail, hard copies of emails, interesting Internet articles you printed to read later - they pile up, and eventually you have to deal with them. Why not use technology?

Try scanning the documents you need to keep and then store them virtually – in the cloud – using something like DropBox (dropbox.com). It's a great place to store any document you don't need in hard copy. Then celebrate when you recycle all that paper!

If you think the cloud isn't safe, store the scanned documents on your computer or on a portable hard drive (that you could keep even safer in a safety deposit box). You will always have access to any document you've saved, and you can print out a hard copy if necessary.

~ Valerie C Krupp

Valerie Krupp, BMEd, MALS, ADHD Coach, helps adult clients put the puzzle pieces of ADHD together to create their best life. ADDultLifeCoaching.com (803) 413-7398

Get a Coach!

One of the best strategies to learn more about the impact ADHD has on your life is to work with an ADHD Coach. A what, you ask?

An ADHD Coach is someone who provides nonjudgmental support and helps you stay focused on your goals, navigate obstacles, keep in action and address key ADHD related challenges such as time awareness, organization, distractibility, self-esteem, planning, etc. A Coach is your motivator, teacher, champion and accountability partner.

In addition, a coach can create structure, offer support, teach skills and strategies to move you closer to your goals, to deepen your self-awareness, better manage your ADHD related challenges and enjoy a more satisfying life.

~Laurie Dupar, PMHNP, RN, PCC

Laurie Dupar, PMHNP, RN, PCC is a trained Psychiatric Nurse Practitioner and 12 year veteran ADHD coach specializing in mentoring and training emerging ADHD Coaches.
www.coachingforadhd.com support@coachingforadhd.com

Motivate with the ADHD Trifecta

"I don't seem to have any motivation."
"I feel like I can't make myself do it."

"If only I could rely on myself to get it done!"

When you have ADHD, it is hard to find the motivation to make yourself get things done. Rather than beating yourself up for your lack of motivation, use the ADHD Trifecta to create your own motivation.

Intentionally apply the three motivational winners of the ADHD Trifecta when you feel stuck:

HIGH INTEREST

• Start with your talents

• Create curiosity

• Micro-change for novelty

• Reward yourself

LOOMING DISASTER

• Create deadlines

• Set timers

• Log progress

• Create a challenge or game

OTHER PEOPLE

• Set up accountability partners

• Enlist a buddy or make an appointment

• Announce intentions

• Delegate tasks

When you are feeling stuck and unmotivated, make your own motivation by employing tactics from the ADHD Trifecta.

~ Casey Dixon, SCAC, BCC, MSEd

Casey Dixon is Success Strategist and ADHD Coach for www.mindfullyadd.com and www.dixonlifecoaching.com, employing a unique focus on science-based, innovative strategies for demand-ridden professionals with ADHD.

Organization Makes the Grade

Many students do A-level work, but do not receive A's because they are disorganized. You can learn these simple habits and get your assignments finished and turned in!

• Have a place where you keep all your school supplies on the main level of the house. A large bin works well for students with lots of stuff.

• When you finish your homework, always return it to the correct folder and backpack immediately.

• Pack everything the night before.

• Go through backpack, binders, and folders weekly so everything is where it belongs.

• Write down homework in a planner every day.

• Plan in advance for long-term assignments. If you need more time, talk to the teacher in advance.

• If you don't have time for breakfast, bring it with you.

• Be patient. Every new habit takes daily practice.

• If needed, get help.

~ Cheryl Fever Gedzelman

Cheryl Gedzelman, President of Tutoring For Success, offers home based tutoring, test prep, and academic coaching in the Washington, DC area. www.TutoringForSuccess.com (703) 390-9220

"Just be yourself.
Let people see the real,
imperfect, flawed, quirky,
weird, beautiful, magical person that
you are."

~ Mandy Hale

The Ultimate Parent's Question

People with ADHD struggle with self-activation, even if it's something they really want to do. What looks like "lack of motivation" is usually masking something that's hard for ADHDers to do.

As a parent, it's hard to remember this, but it's critical. After all, kids really do LOOK like they're being lazy when they won't get up and take care of a simple task or request. But it's NOT easy for them to get activated, and then focus, and then sustain effort, or they'd probably just do it. One simple homework assignment or household chore requires enormous executive function.

So when you ask your child to do something "simple" and are met with resistance, ask yourself: "What part of this might be difficult for them?"

With a little understanding, you can help your kids break simple tasks down into smaller parts, find motivations and activate!

> ~ Diane Dempster & Elaine Taylor-Klaus,
> Co-Founders, ImpactADHD.com

Diane Dempster, MHSA, PCC, CPC and Elaine Taylor-Klaus, PCC, CPCC, the parenting coaches of ImpactADHD.com, the leading online resource for parents of kids with ADHD.

Planned Procrastination

Procrastination seems to be a naughty word. It is blamed for being late, missing deadlines and laziness. What if you could use procrastination to your advantage...and plan for it?

If you tried other strategies and still find procrastinating is the best approach to tasks, work with your brain to make the most of hyper focus and energy. For instance, forego weekly bill paying and instead plan to stay up late on one Friday night per month to get them paid and in the mail. Plan on ignoring boring daily housework, knowing weekend visitors will have you motivated to get the house in order lickety-split.

Planning for procrastination means that you are purposely putting something aside with the plan of doing it later, when you use natural procrastination energy to focus on that task and get it done.

~Laurie Dupar, PMHNP, RN, PCC

Laurie Dupar, PMHNP, RN, PCC is a trained Psychiatric Nurse Practitioner and 12 year veteran ADHD coach specializing in mentoring and training emerging ADHD Coaches.
www.coachingforadhd.com support@coachingforadhd.com

The Biggest Difference?

The dust bunnies are dancing on the tile as you walk by. The piles of papers have somehow doubled their size overnight. The fish tank is so murky you're not sure if there are still any fish swimming around. And you get a surprise call that a friend, the insurance adjuster, or your mother-in-law will be over in an hour.

So what do you do? You could panic and give up before your start. You could run around in a frenzy and start lots of things, and maybe complete a few. You could decide the pencil drawer desperately needs organizing. Or you could ask yourself a question. (Not "Do I have to open the door?") The question is: "What could I do right now that would make the biggest difference?"

It could be that you sweep the papers into an empty laundry basket and put them out of sight to be dealt with later. You might decide to grab the vacuum and a feather duster and do a good-for-now job of cleaning. Or it could be that just getting the dishes off the tables and out of the sink might do the trick.

Sometimes we get into the all-or-nothing perfectionism trap. Either we clean the whole house, we write the entire presentation, we come up with the best plan – or we give up because it just seems impossible. The biggest-difference question is the middle ground between the two extremes and can be asked in a variety of circumstances: last-minute studying for tomorrow's test, planning an impromptu party, preparing for a work presentation, or organizing a trip.

For tomorrow's test, for example, it would be great to have the time to reread the chapters, rewrite notes and answer all the practice problems. But in planning a "good enough" strategy, the answer to the biggest-difference question will come from thinking about what you understand, how you learn, what is likely to be on the test, and what you have done in the past that has provided good results.

The power in the biggest-difference question lies in the pause – giving us the space to stop, think and move into appropriate action. It allows us to move forward without letting overwhelm, perfectionism, or an I-can't-prioritize mindset, stop us in our tracks.

So as you read this, what goal comes to mind? What could you do right now that would make the biggest difference?

~ Roxanne Fouché, ADHD coach and consultant

Roxanne Fouché specializes in strengths-based coaching of bright students and adults with ADHD, weaknesses in executive functioning, and/or learning differences. She also provides consulting for students, families, and schools. Roxanne has extensive experience working with students and adults, assisting them to live well and flourish with ADHD. She has graduate studies in special education, specialized training in life and ADHD coaching and holds both a professional Certificate in Educational Therapy and a Certificate in Positive Psychology. Roxanne regularly presents at regional and national events. For more information, visit www.FocusForEffectiveness.com. Contact her at Roxanne@FocusForEffectiveness.com or (858) 484-4749.

For Your ADHD, Apologize Not!

'Do or do not-there is no try.' Wondering what the immortal words of Master Yoda have to do with not apologizing? Isn't saying 'I'm sorry,' a sign that the force is strong with this one? Shouldn't people say 'I'm sorry' when they're wrong? Absolutely! But is it 'wrong' to be wacky? Heck no!

I am one of those people who says 'I'm sorry' all the time! If you bump into me, I'll tell you 'I'm sorry.' If you get in my car and it's not very clean, I'll tell you 'I'm sorry.' If I cook dinner for you - and I'm not a good cook - I'll tell you 'I'm sorry.' If I bring in take out for dinner, but I think you would've wanted me to cook instead, I'll tell you 'I'm sorry.' If I'm 5 minutes late, I'll tell you 'I'm sorry.' If I'm 5 minutes early, I'll tell you 'I'm sorry I'm early!' It's exhausting! When I was diagnosed with ADHD as an adult, I realized I had spent a lot of time apologizing for the ways my ADHD impacted those around me. I felt like I was always letting people down. You know how this goes - late again, showing up for appointments on the wrong day (if I remember to show up at all) never able to find what I need in the piles around me. I was always 'trying' to do better, to be better.

Getting diagnosed was a huge step towards 'doing,' not just 'trying.' I've found endless ways to manage my ADHD life -

dinner services, paper everything, toiletries by the kitchen sink, hiring my kids to organize the house, to name a few. But imagine this, I still spent an equal amount of time apologizing! This time for my wacky solutions! Not very Jedi Master of me, eh?

So, here's the deal: the wacky ways are only wacky to people who don't get ADHD. For us and ours, wacky ways are lifesavers! Why apologize for something that makes my life better? I admit my first instinct when someone sees the toothbrushes in my kitchen or finds out that I outsource almost everything is still to apologize. I want to say 'I'm sorry I'm still not more organized/responsible/thrifty/etc.' But that's pre-diagnosis me talking. ADHD Jedi Master Proud Me knows that I am using my strengths and gifts in the best way possible! And it's working! So, I stopped apologizing for my wacky ways. And an amazing thing happened! I felt stronger and more capable! The force IS strong with this one! Turns out, all those 'I'm sorrys' take a toll on our self-worth. Definitely not what Yoda wants for us...So, DO resist the urge to apologize when you've found a wacky way that works for you. Do NOT change your life because it doesn't look like someone else's. And always, live long and prosper.

~ Jeremy Didier, AAC

Jeremy Didier, AAC became an ADHD Coach after founding Kansas City's award winning CHADD chapter, ADHDKC. A graduate of both

JST & ADDCA's coaching programs, Jeremy works with parents of ADHD kids, adolescents and young adults with ADHD to create success strategies for the entire family.

Red is the Color of my Heart

Being the mom of a hyperactive and impulsive ADHD son meant that it was a constant challenge to keep my eyes on him, especially when we would go on outings. Not wanting to be a clinging parent and still give my unpredictable child some freedom to spread his wings, I serendipitously came up with a solution. By chance I realized that when he was dressed in red I was quickly able to scan a crowd and find my sweet, adorable, constantly on the go son. For years the primary color of his wardrobe was red: red shirts, red caps, red jacket and even red swim trunks!

To this day I am not sure he realizes that it wasn't eyes in the back of my head that always knew what he was up to, but the color red.

~Laurie Dupar, PMHNP, RN, PCC

Laurie Dupar, PMHNP, RN, PCC is a trained Psychiatric Nurse Practitioner and 12 year veteran ADHD coach specializing in mentoring and training emerging ADHD Coaches.
www.coachingforadhd.com   support@coachingforadhd.com

Buzz Ya Later: Tools to Tame Your Time Optimism

"Just one more thing!" you say. And the next thing you know, you're running behind! Want to stay on top of both your curiosities AND your calendar? Break your day down in reverse – time might expand when you start with the end in mind:

• Assess your time, blocking off commutes and appointments.

• Gather necessary accessories the night before – leave them where they will be lying in wait OR where you will be sure to trip over them!

• Nudge yourself to transition to the next task? Find a tool that fits you best. My FitBit is a vibrational force of subtlety!

• Rule of 3 – Select only 3 items from your master task list for your day.

• Most importantly, resist the urge to add anything 15 minutes before your next "to do" and let your rock star timing propel you from time optimism to time reality.

~ Kate Barrett, ADHD Coach & Parent Educator

Kate Barrett, ADHD Coach and CHADD-certified Parent-to-Parent Educator, specializes in helping you gain perspective on ADHD and navigate your way to personal success. www.coachingcville.com info@coachingcville.com

Finding the Upside to Keep from Getting Down

As a kid, having no "think first button" for my actions often got me into trouble. Medication helped me to control my impulses and think things through before I spoke or acted. However, I started to have different problems with socialization. It was as though all my skill and natural ease for making friends and idle conversation just kind of vanished. As the meds would leave my system the impulsivity part of me started to return. I'm naturally spontaneous, think quickly, am playful and make people smile. This part of what people call "impulsivity" is something that has made me a requested camp counselor for kids at summer camps for years! No longer a burden, it's part of the reason I have made lifelong friends who view my ADHD as a gift.

~ Dr. Billi Bittan

Dr. Billi, PhD, certified Co-active ADHD Coach and Neuro-Cognitive Behavioral Therapist, is the founder of AttentionB and creator of the LEVERAGE ADHD™ System. www.attentionb.com

"Tell me...

what is it you plan to do

with your one wild

and precious life?"

~ Mary Oliver

Follow that Squirrel!

The story of the squirrel in the land of ADHD is globally familiar, but it's what happens when you follow that squirrel that counts!

Movement is vital in working with ADHD brains. Research shows it plays a major role in helping retain information and work out cognitive tasks (Journal of Abnormal Child Psychology). Building movement into homework and study skills is a must when I work with individuals. The more movement strategies, the more they uncover their creativity and discover their own "wacky and fun ways" of studying while moving. Homework can be a HUGE stressor for kids and parents. Movement and fun can change that!

If you follow that squirrel, you may find one of my teens swinging from the branches of a tree while her mom throws out vocabulary words for an upcoming quiz! Who wouldn't want to study in this environment? So, follow that squirrel!

~ Judy A. MacNamee; ADHD Founder/Coach
ADHD CoachConnect

Judy A. MacNamee, certified ADHD coach, works with teens and adults in developing life changing executive function strategies, igniting strengths and confidence! www.adhdcoachconnect.com judy@adhdcoachconnect (614) 804-6706

How to Find an ADHD Coach

Thinking of hiring an ADHD Coach to help you manage your ADHD related challenges, but feel overwhelmed with that first step of finding one?

1. Use the Internet. Coaches are trained to work virtually (by phone or Skype) so you're not limited by skhansen@surewest.net (ACO – www.ADHDcoaches.org) to find a list of trained ADHD coaches. Try a Google search for words like 'coaching for ADHD,' 'ADHD coaching,' or 'ADHD Coach.'

2. Check out their background. Pay close attention to where and how they were trained and if they were certified or credentialed. An easy way to know? See if they have an ACC, PCC or MCC after their name.

3. Meet the coach. Most coaches offer a brief complimentary consultation to see if they are a good fit for you. Share your story and needs and ask them their approach to coaching.

~Laurie Dupar, PMHNP, RN, PCC

Laurie Dupar, PMHNP, RN, PCC is a trained Psychiatric Nurse Practitioner and 12 year veteran ADHD coach specializing in mentoring and training emerging ADHD Coaches.
www.coachingforadhd.com   support@coachingforadhd.com

Why Working In A Noisy Place Actually Works!

Working in silence and serenity has its benefits. But, don't dismiss the possible advantages of working in a noisy environment. It might be time to take your laptop and wrap yourself in racket.

The most overlooked distraction is our thoughts. For those with ADHD it is often the biggest barrier to paying attention. Efforts we make to lessen external distractions don't work for tuning-out our own thoughts.

Music, TV, bright neon lights are distracting to most. For others, those are crucial to keeping focused. What works for the neuro-typical brain does not work for the complex ADHD brain.

When you notice your kids distracted by irrelevant sights and sounds, quickly bouncing from one activity to another, or becoming bored quickly, what do you do?

If you tell your kids, "Go study in your room where it is quiet," you are not alone. I did it; I didn't know better. Other well-meaning parents and experts share this as an effective focusing strategy. It may be for some, but not others.

Why I thought, "Study in your room where it is quiet," was the secret sauce to focusing and getting stuff done for my daughter:

• Works for me!

• Quiet is necessary to concentrate. I learned it in school.

• Her room has all the required ingredients for success with a desk, comfortable yet studious chair, good lighting, and a clock.

Why did this recipe fail?

Things I didn't notice were my daughter's bright, shiny attention stealers in her room, including:

• Colored pencils and markers. First, organizing them. Second, doodling.

• Fears. Specifically, fear of bugs. The bug on the window? Is it inside or outside? Cautious detective work could take hours.

• The chair. What was I thinking? A chair with wheels and spins. Nothing left to say about the chair.

• A clock. Another fear. Fear of time. Ever hear of time blindness? Daylight would turn to night and still no awareness of time.

• Stuck? Stopping to ask me for help? Mostly, the question was forgotten before she found me. Sometimes, she never found me because something more interesting grabbed her attention while en route.

Our New Improved Secret Sauce to Better Focus? The Kitchen Counter.

Smack-dab in the middle of the energy hub of the house. This is where she gets it all done. We don't change a thing. The phone still rings. The TV in the next room is blaring.

Balancing the checkbook, working on the computer, making dinner, it didn't matter what I was doing. Without realizing it, I became her body double.

A body double is someone who is present and passive with another, who isn't doing the same task with that person or for that person. Their passive presence anchors them to the task at hand, helping them stay focused.

If she got stuck, I was there to help. If I noticed frustration creeping in, I'd suggest a break, a glass of water or fresh air.

The activity and noise is chaotic to me. For my daughter, the thoughts flitting frantically in her head is chaotic.

How do those with overactive minds control their distracting thoughts? They focus on the external noise. It brings their racing thoughts to a screeching halt. The external noise drowns out their more distracting internal thoughts allowing them to focus.

The next time you try to formulate a Secret Sauce, get your kid involved in problem solving. Pause before telling your kid what to do. Ask your kid for ideas! You'll be amazed how many answers your child has when given the space to find them.

~ Carlene Bauwens, Certified ADHD Coach

Carlene Bauwens coaches people to silence their inner critic and to start trusting themselves with their own answers so they can confidently do what they want to do and feel successful. As an Certified ADHD Coach and parent, Carlene's mission is to show people how ADHD is really impacting their family, to break the fail-and-punish cycle, and to embrace each other's differences. She works with people of all ages who are ready to move past their ADHD challenges, focus on their strengths and flourish. Check out all of Carlene's great resources on ADHD, executive functions, social skills, and positivity at http://coachcarlene.com

The Focus Formula

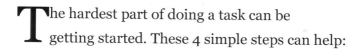

The hardest part of doing a task can be getting started. These 4 simple steps can help:

1. Plan - Decide what you will do, and when you will do it.

2. Set Up - Gather everything you need, and have it ready - separate from the task you will be doing.

3. Sprint - The thought of spending 5 hours on a task probably fills you with dread. So set a timer and work for a 30 minute 'sprint.' Then, take a break if you need it, or keep going if you are focused.

4. Brain Dump - When you walk away from an incomplete task, the chances are that it will feel like starting all over again when you return. So make a note of what you need to do next before you walk away. When you return it will be easier to start on your next sprint.

~ Dr. Michele Toner, PhD, PCC, PCAC

Dr. Michele Toner, PhD, PCC, PCAC, is an ADHD coach. She works with her clients to conquer the chaos and stay in control. www.micheletoner.com

ADHD Writing!?! Wacky Happy
WACKY ADHD

IMPULSIVE

AppySooLutely - Why Not - A Wacky Author

Impulse I – And Off To Dream Thinking I Go

DEADLINES: Two Or Three Junes Away – To Think And Write And Play

Diddly Doing With That Date Of Diddly

RISKS: Plastic Pays My Way – While I Roll Some Dicey Spicy Words

And Work - So Easy Free

RULES: Any And All – Always Read – Any And All – But If I Must

I Will Selfie Twitter And pdfy The z A Booking Face To Space Blog Me

Dream I Will To Think My Way - Authoring Wacky

DAYDREAMS: ??? Out Of My Wacky Mind !!! Very Very Muchly Much

MISSunderSTANDINGS

please remind me once again

?!? when is it you want me to paint the fence !?!

"HAPPINESS Is a journey not a destination" – Father Alfred D'Souza

ADHD writing is my journey of happiness

Minding never the sense nor ever and end

Live the heck out of Your ADHD

and JOURNEY HAPPY

~ Michael Alan Schuler MD

Michael Alan Schuler MD - ADHD Internist Artist Writer - Retirement Celebrating with ECHOES AND SHADOWS CHASING LIGHT - www.woosterbook.com Mike's poems, essays, drawings about any and everything echoesandshadows1212@yahoo.com

"I guess we are who we are for a lot of reasons. And maybe we'll never know most of them.
But even if we don't have the power to choose where we come from, we can still choose where we go from there."

~ Unknown

Get There on Time

Guilty of missing too many dental or medical appointments? I am famous for forgetting those scheduled six months in advance meetings. In fact, when I set the appointment, the receptionist and I place a bet on the chances of my showing up. That is until I set up some simple tools to help me not only remember, but also get to my appointments on time. Before I leave the doctor's office, I do these steps:

1. I put the date into my phone. Then I set a reminder to write it on my wall calendar at home and office.

2. I take a picture of the appointment card so I have the visual reminder.

3. I set a reminder on my phone a week before, day before, morning of and hour before my appointment. I make sure the hour before is a vibrating alarm so I don't miss it.

~Laurie Dupar, PMHNP, RN, PCC

Laurie Dupar, PMHNP, RN, PCC is a trained Psychiatric Nurse Practitioner and 12 year veteran ADHD coach specializing in mentoring and training emerging ADHD Coaches.
www.coachingforadhd.com support@coachingforadhd.com

Skyping Through the House We Go!

Skyping is a fantastic tool for ADHD coaching. I love using this creative method with clients. I support them with time management and organization.

One of my clients struggles with organization. She is very visual, so when she needs to organize her room, we draw a four-square map of her room to chunk it into manageable parts. Then we Skype to get to work! When I'm on screen, she carries me down the hall, past the dog, and her sisters' rooms. I'm sure to say hi to all along the way to her room. When we get to her room, on goes the laptop to show me which quadrant we are focusing on. We have fun while organizing piles of laundry and papers. She takes before and after pictures to see her progress. She says this helps her feel good about her living space.

~ Candace Sahm, MA Ed, JST Coach Training

Candace Sahm, MA Ed, ADHD Coach and Special Educator with JST Coach training. Supports youth and adults to reach their highest potential. 25 years experience.

Communicate Wisely-
With Wacky Words

They say, "choose your words wisely," but how about wacky AND wise? When we get into a heated discussion or an ugly attitude arises with a child, teen or spouse, wise words are often hard to come by, or heard. Both sides can communicate assertively with kindness if they have something to help quickly switch the intensity. This has worked extremely well with my teenage children!

1. Choose to talk in a different voice, like with a foreign accent or that of a favorite cartoon character.

2. Ask the other person to choose and start talking in their favorite voice.

3. Continue the conversation, but listen intently and respond kindly, in your wacky voices. Be ready for some laughter and a better level of connecting. When applied with light-heartedness, it can change the emotional state so that more responsive (wise) words can be chosen, heard and understood by everyone.

~ Melissa R. Fahrney, MA, ACC, CSS

Melissa R. Fahrney, Life Coach and School Psychologist, helps students and adults with ADHD/stress resilience/career development. She recommends daily laughter for "best" self-care. www.labyrinthscoaching.com

The Toilet Paper Test

D o you care how the toilet paper is loaded, bottom or top?

If you do, that's fine. You're entitled to your preference.

But what happens when someone in your family prefers it differently? Do you agree to disagree? When our kids see the world differently from us, we often correct them, instead of respecting their different preference. This adds an extra level of correction that our kids could do without, and takes away their sense of control – and seriously, we want them to start feeling MORE in control, not less!

So if you want your kids to do more around the house, it may be time to stop worrying about whether the laundry is folded just right. If you're not sure if this applies to you, take the toilet paper test: if you REALLY care, it might be a sign that it's time to chill out a little!

~ Diane Dempster & Elaine Taylor-Klaus, co-Founders, ImpactADHD.com

Diane Dempster, MHSA, PCC, CPC and Elaine Taylor-Klaus, PCC, CPCC, the parenting coaches of ImpactADHD.com, the leading online resource for parents of kids with ADHD.

ADHD and Entrepreneurs

I've been an ADHD coach for thirteen years and have been mentoring emerging ADHD coaches for half that time and there is something I have noticed: 99% of ADHD coaches either have ADHD themselves or love a person with ADHD. Either way they have a lot of life experience with this brain style!

I've actually put a name to the common innate talents common to people with ADHD and entrepreneurs...I call it an entrepreneurial brain style. It's true!

In fact people with ADHD are 300% more likely to be entrepreneurs! Both think out-of-the-box, are incredibly creative, have little problem with risk taking, and hyper focus on a task if they are incredibly interested or passionate about it. These natural traits along with many others help us to succeed and do things most people can't even imagine.

What about you? Do you have what it takes to be an ADHD Coach?

~Laurie Dupar, PMHNP, RN, PCC

Laurie Dupar, PMHNP, RN, PCC is a trained Psychiatric Nurse Practitioner and 12 year veteran ADHD coach specializing in mentoring and training emerging ADHD Coaches.
www.coachingforadhd.com   support@coachingforadhd.com

Just One Meaningful Word

A heightened emotional state can intensify our own variety of ADHD behavior. An abrupt change can trigger us, regardless of whether the emotion is good or bad.

I suspect the character Mad Margaret from Gilbert & Sullivan's operetta Ruddigore was misdiagnosed. This exceedingly odd lady's impulsiveness, untidiness, and exuberance were not madness, but my favorite flavors of ADHD! She was thought of as the archetype of all women ... who defy propriety.

To reduce her "madness," Margaret had the clever idea to have her husband use a word with a hidden meaning to calm her whenever he noticed she was about to relapse to odd behavior. It worked. Whenever he said the word, it "recall(ed) her to her saner self."

Find your one word or phrase and make it something that can be uttered in polite company. Whether it is the power of distraction, intention, or awareness, it's effective!

~ *Angelis Iglesias* HSP HSS ADHD Coach
Consultant Researcher

Angelis Iglesias, HSP HSS ADHD, Coach, Researcher Technology, Social Media for Coaches Faculty Impact Coaching Academy
www.mindheartinstitute.com   www.angelisiglesias.com
ai@angelisiglesias.com

ADHD ~ It Can Happen to Anybody!

Recently, I had an intake session with a famous professor from an Ivy League University. Five minutes before the session, his secretary called to let me know he would be 10 minutes late for the call. Exactly 10 minutes after the hour, my phone rang. The first thing this Ivy League professor told me was that he is tired of getting lost! He said, "I've taken this route for the last 15 years, and I get lost two or three times a month! I don't get it!"

I told him I understood why he must be frustrated and said this was a good place to start our coaching. He told me the reason he decided to get a coach was because of an incident at a recent conference. My client left the conference to go to the restroom before his presentation, but got lost in the hotel and couldn't even remember the name of the room! He was supposed to start his talk at 10:00 am and it was already 10:15! He finally saw a colleague, who told him everybody was worried something had happened to him. Of course, my client was embarrassed. But he started laughing at himself and decided to tell this story to start his presentation!

"I know you were all wondering where I was, so I will tell you. I was lost in the hotel! You might not believe me, but I have to admit that sometimes I even get lost in my own complex at home!"

Everybody laughed at his story, and he was able to flow seamlessly into the presentation he prepared for the conference.

After hearing this story, I explained to my client the relationship between ADHD and Executive Functioning, and he told me that this is exactly what he experiences! He said his Executive Functioning skills are absent! Not only does he get lost, but his desk is a mess, he loses important papers all the time, and forgets appointments at least once a week.

I asked him how many secretaries he has and he told me just one! Then I asked him about his wife. He told me that his wife was his exact opposite and takes care of all the details he had trouble paying attention to. I asked him whether he would consider his wife his Executive Secretary to make up for his Executive Functioning challenges? He laughed and said he never thought about it that way, but it sure makes sense and he thinks he owes his success mainly to his wife for taking care of all the things he isn't good at. We were both laughing at that point and I told him I'm sure his wife needed a bit of a break, and he should continue working with his strengths, but also learn some tools to help improve his Executive Functioning to take some of the pressure away from his wife.

My client said he has one secret tool he uses - humor. He always laughs at himself, when he is alone and with others. He said humor is the one thing that has helped lessen the shame he feels about all the basic tasks he has a hard time with! It decreases his anxiety and alleviates the frustration that builds up when he can't figure something out.

And now, what does he do when he speaks at a conference? He tells everybody what happened to him that day. And, if he needs to use the restroom in the middle of conference, he always asks a volunteer to follow him!

~ Roya Kravetz, PCC, BCC, CMC, CPE

Roya Kravetz is a Board Certified and ICF Credentialed Life Coach specializing in strength-based coaching for children, teens, adults, and parents whose lives are affected by ADHD or similar behavioral and/or organizational challenges. She is also a certified Career Coach, mainly for clients with an ADHD diagnosis. Roya is Co-Founder and a Thought-Leader for Parenting 2.0, an international movement that facilitates positive change by nurturing a more proactive life skills educational process. She has been published several times and is a regular speaker at local, national and international conferences. Fluent in three languages, Roya coaches clients nationally and internationally.www.adhdsuccesscoaching.com

Smile To Focus

Smiling is powerful. It signals the brain's reward center to release "feel good" neurotransmitters like Dopamine and Serotonin that trigger happiness and motivation. ADHDers often have to work harder to trigger the brain's reward center, so this simple strategy is great news! When I took the 4+ hour Graduate Record Exam, I made a conscious decision to smile when I arrived in the exam room. It boosted my confidence, I felt more relaxed, and most importantly, I was able to focus on the task at hand. Prior to the exam, I had also utilized a study group, practice tests, tutoring, a prep course, the long process to get needed accommodations...and I practiced smiling throughout all of it! In the end, as someone who has never performed well on standardized tests, it was the smiling that helped me focus at the moment it was needed most. Did you smile today?

~ Ariel Davis, ADHD Coach

Ariel Davis, ADHD Coach/Occupational Therapy Master's Candidate, uses her experience with dual-diagnosed teens/adults and the creative arts to discover and build client strengths.
www.ADHDstrengthscoach.com ADHDstrengthscoach@gmail.com

"Be weird.

Be random.

Be who you are.

Because you never know who would

love the person you hide."

~ Unknown

Lazy Susan Homework

Do you find asking your child to sit down and pay attention doesn't work to get homework done? You might try the "Lazy Susan Homework" method!

Clear a large space like a dining table, bed or floor. Make sure there is plenty of room for your child to move around.

Next, have your child arrange the homework assignments by putting different pieces at different "stations" around the area - science project is at the head of the table, math at the other end.

Finally, have your child set a timer for 10 minutes and start anywhere...it doesn't matter where. When the timer rings, have your child move to the next station and reset the timer to begin the new subject, project, or task.

Continue around, resetting the timer, until all the homework is complete!

~Laurie Dupar, PMHNP, RN, PCC

Laurie Dupar, PMHNP, RN, PCC is a trained Psychiatric Nurse Practitioner and 12 year veteran ADHD coach specializing in mentoring and training emerging ADHD Coaches.
www.coachingforadhd.com support@coachingforadhd.com

That's It! Room, Game, Snack!

Are you forever arguing with your child and feeling like it's going nowhere? He's yelling and angry and won't listen to a word you're saying. Not only is this frustrating, it's fruitless! Why? Because with all the anger and emotion flying around, the CEO of the brain (those Executive Function Skills) has been hijacked by the Amygdala (the part of the brain associated with feelings of fear and aggression).

Without Calm, there is NO learning, reasoning, or problem solving!

So next time your child is stuck in anger mode and you can't reach him, break the negative current and suggest a snack and a short game (ex. Connect 4, Mastermind, Uno). Then as the mood softens you will have a better opportunity to discuss the problem calmly.

~ Cindy Goldrich, EdM, ACAC

Cindy Goldrich, EdM, ACAC, is an ADHD Parent Coach, Teacher Trainer, and author of 8 Keys to Parenting Children with ADHD. www.PTScoaching.com Cindy@PTScoaching.com (516) 802-0593

Fifty Shades of Grey

Recently I was running a workshop for adults with ADHD on the topic of planning, and I was having difficulty convincing my audience that "plan" is not just another four-letter word.

Janet calmly told me she would never, ever plan again. You see, every time she planned her week, things went perfectly well for a time, and then the plan stopped working and she just went back to being her disorganized self. She had decided she was great at designing plans, but was incapable of sticking to them.

Bill identified with her dilemma. He had given up on planning his days at work, because each time he went to the trouble of plotting out what he would do, he was unable to get it all done. He knew he was incapable of designing an effective plan and had given up trying. So planning was a waste of time, right? Heads nodded in agreement

I pointed out to the group that Janet and Bill had shared examples of Black and White Thinking, and I invited them all to step with me into the grey. Shock and horror ensued. Surely there was only one way to do things? And everyone knows people with ADHD can't stick to plans. And besides, grey is such a 'nothing' color! "Rumor has it," I informed them, "that there are 50 Shades of Grey."

Suddenly I had their undivided attention, and we started to play in those shades of grey. Janet's shade of grey enabled her to acknowledge that she could build on her short successes and devise ways of modifying her plans when they became less effective. Bill played with a different shade of grey until he had an "aha" moment. Although he was bad at planning, he was indeed an expert on what he needed to get done at work. He could work with someone, like an ADHD coach, to translate his expertise into a plan that he could test-drive, until he found something that worked for him.

So, next time you find yourself thinking in terms of "all or nothing" and "never or always," remind yourself that Black and White Thinking will not solve your problem. Instead, take your inventive, resourceful brain for a play in the grey – all fifty shades of it.

~ Michele Toner, PhD, PCC, PCAC

Dr. Michele Toner, PhD, PCC, PCAC, is based in Western Australia, and coaches people from around the world. Her Masters and PhD research, coupled with 20 years of hands-on experience make her well equipped to empower her clients, as they learn to conquer the chaos and stay in control. She works with individuals and their families to identify and harness their strengths, address their challenges, and make ADHD 'work for them.' As a registered mentor coach, Michele also empowers new coaches to be the best they can be. www.micheletoner.com

A Wacky Way to Think Clearly

G rab a pencil or a pen – or even a chopstick ...and put it between your teeth. Not outward like a cigar, but gripped across your teeth, like you're biting into it...

Go ahead. I'll wait.

This forces what's called a Duchenne smile – where your whole face is affected. Note how your cheeks force your eye lines to crinkle. That's a Duchenne smile. Now, take that thing out of your mouth and scream, "Thanks Alan!"

Because research shows induced smiling makes you happier, increases your enjoyment of things, and may benefit your heart. (Only the big, Duchenne smile garners these benefits.)

Smiling reduces your stress response, regardless of whether you actually feel happy or not. Reduced stress helps maintain oxygen in the brain and therefore helps us THINK; and another thing smiling does, is increase serotonin production, which is a key neurotransmitter we ADDers depend on for focus.

Now say, "Cheeeeeese!"

~ Alan Brown

Alan Brown, entrepreneur and ADHD coach, created ADD Crusher™ videos and interactive tools that help ADDers live to their potential. Get his free eBook: www.ADDCrusher.com

"Be a Fruit Loop in a world of Cheerios."

~ Unknown

Found It. It's in My Pants!

One of the funniest stories my friend with ADHD ever told me was how she found the key when she got locked out of her car. You'll see why I admire her when I tell you this story!

This wasn't the first time she had been locked out of the car, as the many dents and pry marks made clear. A friend of hers was just about to break in when an observant bystander named "Papa Jim" told her the key was in the waistband of her pants.

Someone later asked my friend if she found her key. With her characteristic unchecked exuberance, she replied, "Yes, Papa Jim found it down my pants!"

Anybody would feel embarrassed, right? Not my friend – her reaction was "OK, I have another amusing story to share with people!" Now that's seeing the bright side! I'd like to be more like my friend!

~ Dr. Kari Miller, PhD, BCET

Dr. Kari Miller, ADHD coach and educational therapist, helps women focus and organize so they get more done and finish what they start! www.ADHDclearandfocused.com Kari.Miller.coach@gmail.com

Considering Becoming an ADHD Coach?

H ere are some interesting facts that show how necessary ADHD coaches will be in the very near future:

- There are over 300 million people with ADHD worldwide. Coaches, trained to work with clients over the phone, can reach into far corners of the world and help these people with ADHD.

- Many people aren't fully diagnosed until their late 50s or 60s, often after they see the ADHD behaviors in their grandchildren. This population is seeking out ADHD coaches in increasing numbers.

- ADHD coaching is now endorsed by top leaders and organizations in the ADHD community as a valuable method to help people with ADHD better manage their challenges. That endorsement leads to visibility and credibility of ADHD coaching, which means more people will be looking to work with an ADHD coach.

Yes, it's an exciting time to be an ADHD coach!

~Laurie Dupar, PMHNP, RN, PCC

Laurie Dupar, PMHNP, RN, PCC Psychiatric Nurse Practitioner and 12 year veteran ADHD coach specializes in mentoring and training emerging ADHD Coaches. www.IACTCenter.com

The LEGO Meltdown

"It's too much, Mom. I'll never be able to do it!" Those were the frustrated, heartfelt, tear stained words from, Carlton, my 13-year-old son.

I had just given him a written list of tasks he needed to complete. And there was one that caused the ADHD meltdown. Item #3: "PICK UP ALL THE LEGOS AND PUT THEM IN THE BASKET." For over a week I had been patient as I stepped over the precious piles in his room because he was "working on a project." However, we were leaving town the next day and it was time to clear the LEGO rubble.

A few years ago, I would have just expected him to do it. When he couldn't, I would get frustrated, lose my cool and blow my top. None of which helped and only made the situation worse. Back then I didn't understand that ADDers are easily overwhelmed. For me, when I looked at the pile of LEGOS in Carlton's room, my brain quickly decided on an action plan and broke the task into manageable steps. In contrast my son's ADHD brain gets overwhelmed and shuts down. His brain only saw a bedroom floor scattered with LEGOS and no possible way to clean them up. What I understand now is that the intensity at which Carlton reacted to the pile of LEGOS was an outward manifestation of the intensity he was feeling inside.

So how did we handle the LEGO meltdown? First, I stayed calm by reminding myself this was a neurological reaction, not a behavioral problem. Next, I took him out of the space and softly told him it was OK and we would get through this together. I also stayed with him and talked him through the process of cleaning up the LEGO piles. Finally, when we were finished, I retraced our steps and said, "That wasn't so bad. Did you see how we broke it down and accomplished it fairly quickly?"

Although my hope was that he would take care of the LEGO piles on his own, it was only when I adjusted MY expectations that we were able to complete the task and organize the LEGOS in the basket. Occasionally I still lose my patience, but learning to adjust my expectations allows me to be patient with my ADDer and myself and minimize the dreaded LEGO meltdowns!

~ Jennifer E. Kampfe, MS

Jennifer Kampfe, MS is an emerging ADHD Coach currently training to become a certified coach. Mother of five, with two sons diagnosed with ADHD, Jennifer is familiar with the challenges faced by both parents and children living with Attention Deficit. Located in Lincoln, NE she looks forward to sharing her ADHD experience and expertise as a resource to the community, offering encouragement, education, support and coaching to parents, children and teens. Visit her website and blog at www.fantasticallyfocused.com. Jennifer may be reached via email at fantasticallyfocused@gmail.com or by phone (402) 613-6646. Like her Facebook page at https://www.facebook.com/fantasticallyfocused.

Birds of a Feather

It's really helpful to spend time with other people with ADHD, as they are more likely to "get" us, whether it's in an ADHD-friendly family gathering, a support group or a group of spirited friends. It allows us to realize that we are not alone, provides unconditional acceptance, corroborates our view of the world, and gives us a sense of joyful community. In addition, it also offers opportunities for great conversations about how to flourish with ADHD. We can forget someone's name, lock ourselves out of our car, go off on a tangent, or lose track of the conversation - and it's okay. We are within a community of equals, each with our own gifts and quirks, appreciating and supporting each other. So check out local or online ADHD support groups, look into ADHD-related MeetUps, or get together with like-minded people. Birds of a feather soar together!

~ *Roxanne Fouché, ADHD coach and consultant*

Roxanne Fouché, strengths-based ADHD coach and consultant, assists students and adults live well and flourish with ADHD. Contact her at Roxanne@FocusForEffectiveness.com or (858) 484-4749.

"And above all,

watch with glittering eyes

the whole world around you because

the greatest secrets

are always hidden

in the most unlikely places.

Those who don't believe in magic

will never find it."

~ Roald Dahl

Counting Goals in Days

Who knew that thinking about upcoming goals in terms of days rather than months or years motivates action? Counting months, rather than years, has a beneficial effect when trying to reach a goal.

This trick, discovered by Professor Daphna Oyserman of the University of Southern California, makes you feel closer to reaching a goal so you start four times sooner!

Whether it is saving for retirement, working on a term paper or starting an exercise routine, thinking in terms of the number of days to achieve the goal was more motivating.

So next time you want to change a habit, reach a new milestone or have a long term project to complete, thinking of it in terms of the number of days (or months) it will take to complete, will have you starting and finishing it easier and sooner!

~Laurie Dupar, PMHNP, RN, PCC

Laurie Dupar, PMHNP, RN, PCC is a trained Psychiatric Nurse Practitioner and 12 year veteran ADHD coach specializing in

mentoring and training emerging ADHD Coaches.
www.coachingforadhd.com   support@coachingforadhd.com

SPINNING TOP SPINNING COLORS

??? Imagine That !!!

Oh My Oh My - So Much Sense Now I See

Embraced Did I The Spinning Top That Was Spinning My Me

Sixty Five Nearly I Am - Years Not Months

And ADHD He Is Telling Me I Be

OK --- OK --- Okaaay - What The Heck

The Chancy Stuff Chancing I Like

Give Me Those ADHD Glasses

Let Me See What I Can See Of Myself

The Life That Was And Is The Life Of Me

Like So Many Of The Rest Of You And Me

Born I Was A Colorful Spinning Top

Into This World Of Gray Which Plods Along

Straight And Narrow - Blinders On

Loving Did I To Play The Playful Play

Playing Deep Deep Inside Of Me

But In Those Early Days Of Me

The Days Were Rained By Gray

And So It Was At Ten Years Not Months

A Reckoning Talk Occurred Within My Depths So Deep

I Took To Wearing Their Gray - Found Some Blinders

And Best I Could Took Aim To Spin Narrow And Straight

One Hell Of A Time We Have Had - My ADHD And Me

Color Spinning Pretending Gray On Their Straight And
Narrow Way

Tales And Stories And Stories And Tales

Far Beyond Any Telling I Could Tell Here

But Let Me Give You This Little Taste

A Thousand Women I Have Loved A Thousand Times And
More

Each And Every - Pat O'Dea - The Light Of My Life

An Imagine For Real Far Beyond Any Imagine That

Color Spinning My Way On The Straight Narrow Gray

Came At A Very Costly Cost

Energy By The Tons I Have Had To Spend

Living So Doing - Never Did I "Think"

My Energy Bank Would Ever Come Up Empty

At Fifty Nine Years Not Months

My Bank Of Energy Closed Its Doors

Sputtering Splintering Toppling Screaming Hollering

I Was Wrenched From A Hell Of A Life Into A Life Of Hell

I Spun Myself Out Of Control

I Came To Know Without Knowing

My ADHD Yet Not ADHD

For I Could Not Completely Convince Myself Nor Anyone Else

And So I Spun Ever Deeper Into A Dance Of Woe And Whine

Caring And Sharing For And With Me

She Did What She Always Has

Guiding Me Back To Light

He Hugged Me And He Loved Me

And ADHD He Told Me I Be

Firing My Fire To Color Spin Again My Me

Being told at sixty four years of age that I am ADHD

Has been intensely empowering and insightful

To help guide myself and my health care efforts

I am utilizing this new found energy to journey a fuller life

In so doing I hope to spin as free as I can without crashing

Bringing color and joy not only to myself but to as many others as I might

I will now embrace my ADHD

Not as Attention Deficit Hyperactivity Disorder

But as ATTENTION DIFFERENT HIGHLY DRIVEN

Although the faces of our ADHD are enormously varied

We do share the trait of immense creative talent

The nature of that talent is unique to each one of us

And that is what makes each one of us extraordinary

I believe that every life is extraordinary

Yours – Mine – Theirs – Every ADHD – No Exceptions

In turn, Heart and Soul

YOU ARE EXTRAORDINARY

Believe in yourself

Find your extraordinary talent

PLEASE – PLEASE – PLEASE I KNOW IT

Let yourself know how extraordinarily wonderful you are

live your life extraordinary

Thanks For Letting Me Color Spin

Whose "talent" is to paint

And M(em) A(ae)

With written words, brushed acrylics and routered wood

Imagine That? Emae

~ *Michael Alan Schuler MD*

Michael Alan Schuler, MD, A Colorful Spinning Top - Attention Different Highly Driven - A former Cleveland Clinic Wooster, Ohio - Internist, Pulmonologist, Intensivist. He remains in Wooster - Celebrating his retirement years With Pat - The Life who allows him the privilege of being her husband. He thinks of himself as an Artist and Writer; ECHOES AND SHADOWS CHASING LIGHT Is a colorful spin of some of his unique views on Life, Family, Health, America, God, ADHD and who knows what else. He is still trying to figure it out. (2012 The Wooster Book Company, Ohio - www.woosterbook.com) echoesandshadows1212@yahoo.com

ADHD Hometown Heroines

I am proud to know many individuals who have ADHD. Two women with whom I have become friends inspire me with their generosity, resilient spirit, and tenacity in the face of obstacles. It doesn't get any more successful than the gifts these inspiring women give the world.

In her role as an intervention specialist at the UCLA children's cancer clinic, Dr. Patty Kerrigan watched heartbroken as many children recovered from cancer only to have significant learning problems brought on by the very treatments that saved their lives. While radiation, chemotherapy and surgery are necessary; in many cases they can diminish children's learning ability.

Her strong desire to help children struggling to succeed in school spurred Dr. Kerrigan to create Foundation ThinkAgain, a non-profit organization that provides remedial therapies to children who are fighting to thrive after cancer.

Dr. Kerrigan struggled in school herself and was diagnosed with ADHD later in life. Although she finds it hard to pay attention and concentrate, she credits ADHD with giving her the gift of the ability to see interesting angles and creative solutions that others do not always see.

Linda Larson Schlitz has been blazing trails all her life! With a master's degree in guidance and counseling, she created and led programs for teens recovering from drug abuse and food addiction. Her many awards include a commendation from the governor of Wisconsin, the Red Cross Hometown Hero award, and the prestigious Athena award given for assisting women in developing professional and leadership skills.

When the state of Wisconsin closed much-needed treatment programs for individuals struggling with alcohol and drug abuse, Linda and her family founded Randlin Adult Family Care Homes, a non-profit organization that assists homeless veterans and adults with mental health issues who have been turned away by other agencies as "untreatable."

Linda's non-profit operated four homes with a total of forty-six beds, giving residents a new start on life. Her mission has always been to help people bring out their unique talents and live a purposeful and independent life. She shares her inspirational gifts in her latest book, which chronicles her ups and downs as a woman with ADHD and Type II Bipolar.

These women embody the sensitivity, inspirational drive, and single-minded pursuit of a goal so characteristic of women with ADHD. Hats off to all ADHD hometown heroines!

~ Dr. Kari Miller, PhD, BCET

Dr. Kari Miller, ADHD coach and board certified educational therapist, helps women conquer their biggest ADHD challenges. She assists women in getting focused, organized, and motivated so they get unstuck, finish what they start, and accomplish more every day! Dr. Miller leverages her expertise as a learning specialist to help women find unique and exciting strategies for managing their ADHD challenges. Through her group and individual coaching programs and online supportive community, she encourages and inspires women to set their sights high and make big changes in their lives! For more information visit www.ADHDclearandfocused.com or www.ADHDcoachingforwomen.com

Kitchens are for Brushing Teeth!

If you visit my house on a school day morning, you will find toothbrushes and toothpaste wedged between the butcher block and the spice rack in the kitchen. You may find this baffling: Are we developing new recipes involving mint and fluoride? Are we using our toothbrushes as vegetable scrubbers? Do we not have bathrooms? The simple truth is this: we brush our teeth at the kitchen sink! As an ADHD Mom with 5 kids, 2 of whom also have ADHD, I struggle with getting everyone (including me!) out the door on time. If my ADHD kids successfully make it to the kitchen wearing something resembling school clothes, the last thing I want to do is send them back upstairs to brush their teeth. An infinite number of distractions lie between the kitchen and the nearest bathroom sink! So, we brush on our way out the door! Wacky, but it works!

~ Jeremy Didier, AAC

Jeremy Didier, ADHD Coach, founder & group coordinator of Kansas City's award winning CHADD chapter-ADHDKC, & ADHD mom of the fabulous five!

When You Love Someone with ADHD

When one half of a relationship has ADHD, small adjustments in communication and expectations can make a world of difference.

1. Decide how to remind. Whether you post, text, call or communicate in person, make sure the inevitable reminder is known to be supportive, loving and nonjudgmental, not nagging.

2. Be clear and concrete in your communication. Set specific times for dates, dinner and when coming home.

3. Before you launch into emotional discussions, ask if the other person is available to listen. This 'availability' means that the other person is in a place to focus and attend to what is being said.

4. Keep a list of the positive qualities of your partner's ADHD so you are reminded of what you enjoy when it feels like their ADHD causes issues in the relationship.

~Laurie Dupar, PMHNP, RN, PCC

Laurie Dupar, PMHNP, RN, PCC is a trained Psychiatric Nurse Practitioner and 12 year veteran ADHD coach specializing in mentoring and training emerging ADHD Coaches. www.coachingforadhd.com support@coachingforadhd.com

"Learn to love the fool in you, the one who feels too much, talks too much, takes too many chances, wins sometimes and loses often, lacks self control, loves and hates, hurts and gets hurt, promises and breaks promises, laughs and cries.

It alone protects you against that utterly self-controlled, masterful tyrant whom you also harbor and who would rob you of human aliveness, humility and dignity but for your fool."

~ Theodore Isaac Rubin

ADHD Color Blind Celebrating

Echoed And Shadowed, Straights And Narrows

ADHD And Color Blind

Life This Lost Finding, Finding Lost

I Zig Zag, Dance Their Black And White

Color Master My Michelangelo's

I Bope Live This Biper World

Discover Finding, Finding Discover

Celebrating My Different Me

Extraordinary every life is. There are no exceptions. Me and You and Every,

We are all each extraordinary. Embrace your extraordinary life and never stop

celebrating it.

To think within the confines of established norms – focused attention

To think outside of the confines of established norms – unfocused attention

Biper/Bipe – a brain inside of the box person

Boper/Bope – a brain outside of the box person.

~ *Michael Alan Schuler MD*

Michael Alan Schuler MD - ADHD Internist Artist Writer - Retirement
Celebrating with ECHOES AND SHADOWS CHASING LIGHT -
www.woosterbook.com - poems, essays, drawings -
echoesandshadows1212@yahoo.com

Hypnotize Yourself to Peace of Mind!

Finding a relaxation technique that energizes us can seem like an impossible quest. These techniques tend to add to our busy agenda. Rather, we want the feeling of relief and peace of mind. Autogenic Training (AT), a form of self-hypnosis, might be the thing you've been looking for!

AT works well for the impatient, fast minded individual. It's easy to learn, can be practiced almost anywhere, the results come quickly and it doesn't require a lot of time each day. AT is also extensively researched and proven effective.

AT involves learning some mental exercises (sentences) focusing on various parts of the body, i.e. "My arms are heavy and warm," "My heart is calm and steady." By passively creating mental contact with these parts, the mind and body can switch off the 'fight/flight' stress response, and promote rest and recovery. AT increases concentration, focus, reduces anxiety and provides a self-empowerment tool.

~ Anna Maria Lindell

Anna Maria Lindell, founder of Advance and ADD Coach Academy graduate, helps entrepreneurs and high achievers with ADHD/ADHD-traits understand their brain, and increase productivity. www.advancesweden.se

Jump Start Motivation

It's often a challenge to get motivated enough to start (and complete) things. Motivation is situational and specific to different tasks and settings. Here are five tips to jump start motivation:

• WHAT: Set a clear intention for what you want to do – and what you will not do.

• WHY: Focus on the meaning of the task, and why it's important to you or someone else.

• WHEN: Plan to work on difficult tasks when you are at your best, in sync with your energy highs.

• WHERE: Visualize where you are going to accomplish the task (your desk? a coffee shop? on the treadmill?).

• HOW: Choose how to start (easiest or hardest thing?); remember past successes; increase novelty and variety; plan for exercise breaks; don't wait until you feel inspired; build in accountability; give yourself rewards; and if you lose focus, start again – as often as necessary!

~ Roxanne Fouché, ADHD coach and consultant

Roxanne Fouché, strengths-based ADHD coach and consultant, assists students and adults live well and flourish with ADHD.
www.FocusForEffectiveness.com/blog
Roxanne@FocusForEffectiveness.com (858) 484-4749

Stop Feeling Guilty and Take A Nap

Napping is wasted on the young. Half the time they'd rather not be doing it. Many adults welcome a good nap, but feel guilty for taking one. In our busy, type-A society, napping has gotten a bad rap.

Focusing hour after hour at work and school is challenging for some and leads to physical and mental exhaustion. Think of the brain as a cell phone battery. Use your cell phone all day and the battery needs to be re-charged.

Napping boosts your mood, alertness, creativity, memory, and performance. It reduces stress and clarifies decision-making.

If it's not too late in the day, you can reap all these benefits with a short nap of 20-30 minutes without interfering with your nighttime sleep.

Instead of thinking about "nappers" as lazy, unambitious souls who slack off, let's consider how self-aware they are to know when they need a break to be their best.

~ Carlene Bauwens, Certified ADHD Coach

Carlene Bauwens, Certified ADHD Coach and parent, empowers teens and adults to focus on their strengths and flourish with ADHD. coachcarlene.com support@coachcarlene.com

"Believe in yourself and all that you are. Know that there is something inside you that is greater than any obstacle."

~ Christian D. Larson

Popsicle Stick Chores

Doing daily chores can often become a boring task for children with ADHD. Boring = not getting done! To help make it a bit more exciting, I write each chore on a Popsicle stick and put it in a "what's next?" jar. Each morning, my children would be eager to see which "chore" they would be doing next based on what stick they pulled. As each stick was pulled and chore completed, they would mark it off until all were done! Sticks went back into a special "done" cup to get ready for tomorrow.

~Laurie Dupar, PMHNP, RN, PCC

Laurie Dupar, PMHNP, RN, PCC is a trained Psychiatric Nurse Practitioner and 12 year veteran ADHD coach specializing in mentoring and training emerging ADHD Coaches.
www.coachingforadhd.com support@coachingforadhd.com

Stop Interruptions and Teach Patient Waiting

We all know that impulsivity and interruptions are a big challenge for kids. This will work (ages 4 to adult)!

1. Teach your child to put her hand on your arm to get your attention when you are busy.

2. Put your hand on her hand to let her know she'll get your attention soon.

3. As quickly as possible, briefly turn your attention to your child.

4. Listen to what she wants to tell you (remind her to keep it simple).

5. Ask her to wait, and return briefly to your original activity.

6. Again, as soon as possible, turn your attention back to your child. This time, either address the issue, or set up a clear time when you will.

This may sound complicated, but it's really quite simple. Gradually teach your kids to wait patiently, little bits at a time.

~ Diane Dempster & Elaine Taylor-Klaus, Co-Founders, ImpactADHD.com

Diane Dempster, MHSA, PCC, CPC and Elaine Taylor-Klaus, PCC, CPCC, parenting coaches of ImpactADHD.com, the leading online resource for parents of kids with ADHD.

Changing the Game Plan – Becoming Good Enough

I learned an insightful strategy from one of my students, "Melissa." She's a collegial student of engineering and psychology and an 'ever optimistic' person. The first time I met her, she was wearing unmatched socks. This pattern continued throughout our sessions so I finally asked her why? She replied that it is one of her unique strategies, to train her executive functions to work for her own personal needs.

Working on how to be "good enough" for each individual can be challenging, especially when outside forces tell you things need to be done a certain way. There are things you can do to help guide you into being enough. For example, when Melissa does laundry she has three baskets: one for clothes, one for undergarments and one for socks. After you wash your socks, according to Melissa, they don't all need to match—they just need to provide the purpose that socks do. There is no need to stress if your socks don't match. I apply a similar tactic in that I don't waste time to fold; I just choose a pair of socks. For me, it's good enough that they stay unfolded and clean. If you are stressed because your socks don't match, buy the same kind.

When you find yourself down and dealing with struggles that accompany having ADHD, remember all the unique and wonderful quirks you have. Write them down. Put them on the mirror so when you look at your reflection the words are there. When you are beating yourself up over what you don't like about yourself, remember all the qualities you do like. When we have ADHD, we can easily get overwhelmed when things aren't going as planned. When we wake up we can either have a peaceful day or a stressful one. We can stress over that matching sock or just be satisfied our feet are warm and covered. What do you choose?

~ Dr. Billi Bittan

Billi Bittan, MA, PhD, is an ADHD Neuro-Cognitive Behavioral / Expressive Arts Therapist and ADHD Coach. Her Los Angeles private practice, AttentionB, specializes in innovative therapy/coaching for ADHD. With 35 years experience in physical education, pedagogy and expressive therapies, she developed the Leverage ADHD™ System to empower others to transform ADHD symptoms and challenges into useful assets. She is the author of the Kindle book "Be the Chief Executive of Your Executive Functions: The Entrepreneurial Way to Leverage ADHD to Your ADDvantage™." Dr. Billi has co-authored numerous books. Visit www.attentionb.com or contact drbilli@attentionb.com. 855-372-4554 (DRBILLI)

The Secret of Connection

What gets in the way of us connecting with our ADHD kids? Connection is one of the best ways to help a child who is struggling with the impulsivity of ADHD. It allows us to help them find regulation when they may be dysregulated. Connecting means being intentional about how we interact with our kids. Looking for opportunities to create a more meaningful bond. How? Look for little things. Share jokes, snuggle, play catch, teach a new skill, learn a new skill from your child. These are just a few ways. Maybe you're already doing one or more of these, but just need to see them as a way of connecting. Connection is the way that your child will sense empathy in the tough times and follow your lead in feeling safe and loved when they are upset. Those small things will pay off in the end.

~ Jared and DeAnn Jennette, Parent Coaches

Jared and DeAnn Jennette are trained coaches who specialize in families of adopted children with ADHD, SPD, and other "alphabet soup" diagnoses. www.embraceparentcoaching.com embraceparentcoaching@gmail.com

Let Freedom Ring, Not the Phone!

Many things happen during the day that can distract us, preventing us from accomplishing our priorities. Answering calls every time the phone rings is a common distracter! Try these four steps:

1. Don't answer your phone. When your phone rings, think of it as someone else's priority . With caller ID, texting, answering machines and voice mail, you really won't miss important messages.

2. Let the "machine" answer. If you are worried you'll miss an emergency call from a loved-one, design an alert system, such as calling twice in a row.

3. Set your phone(s) on silent, and turn off the vibration feature, during your productivity times.

4. Finally, decide and plan ahead when you will listen to messages and return calls.

Following these steps puts your chosen priorities back on top of your schedule where they belong!

~Laurie Dupar, PMHNP, RN, PCC

Laurie Dupar, PMHNP, RN, PCC is a trained Psychiatric Nurse Practitioner and 12 year veteran ADHD coach specializing in mentoring and training emerging ADHD Coaches. www.coachingforadhd.com support@coachingforadhd.com

"It's okay to be scared.

Being scared means you're about to

do something really, really brave."

~ Unknown

The Duplicated (ADHD) Life

Duplicates are a great ADHD coping strategy!

Reading glasses: Buy a dozen cheap readers and stash them all over the house.

Clothes hampers: Buy one for each kind of laundry to save sorting time (blacks, colors, delicates, bras, jeans, etc.)

Makeup/toiletries: Three sets are essential, one for the bathroom, one for the office and one for the car or travel.

Kitchen utensils used constantly, e.g. measuring spoons and cups, have multiples so you don't have to stop to wash them.

Clocks: One or more in every room keeps you aware of time.

Tools and supplies in the glove compartment of <u>each</u> vehicle (utility knife, tissues, tire gauge, reading glasses, screwdrivers, flashlight, dry snacks, pen, Post-Its)

Anything you use and lose often – camera lens cover, nail file, even sets of car keys. It's not expensive to create duplicates, takes up little room and saves SO much grief!

~ Linda Roggli, PCC

Linda Roggli, PCC, helps stop the madness for midlife ADHD women through startlingly effective coaching, transformational retreats and weekend intensives. You ready?
http://addiva.net linda@addiva.nethttp://addivaretreats.com

Making Space for Original Thinking

When I'm stuck in serious procrastination, I physically move whatever's not nailed down out of my office. For a few days, I walk past it. Then, one by one, I vote "survivors" back in. Piles of must read articles and treasured memorabilia that I no longer even see – nothing is spared.

Like too snug clothing inhabiting my closet leading me to believe that if I try harder, I'll find more than the two uniforms I wear daily, these bins of articles and post-its masquerade as brilliant ideas that I must read and ponder thoughtfully.

Creative impulse propels me to collect stuff. But scarcity whispers that I need all of it because what if I toss the pile and miss the one profound word or thought I'm missing?

The process brings me back to center and I exhale knowing I'll be just fine without reading 64 social media articles.

~ Sherri Dettmer Cannon

Sherri Cannon, Executive Coach, ADHD Coach and seasoned workshop leader, helps individuals and teams around the world thrive by leveraging strengths, collaboration and innovation. www.sherricannon.com

Did Curiosity Kill Kat?
Or Give New Life?

It all started when I awoke in the middle of the night. I was a sophomore in college, half way through second semester, and needed to choose a major for my junior year. My university was small, around 2500 students, and conservative. It was right around the time that Kent State happened, so many students nationwide were protesting. Many schools cancelled exams, except my school. I was feeling a little confined. I had this gnawing feeling that there MUST BE something else beyond my college campus.

So my journey to see the world began, if only for a summer, to help me decide between social work and theatre arts. Very soon after my nighttime awakening, I noticed a flyer on a bulletin board that said 'Summer Jobs in Germany.' Here was my answer. I grabbed a flyer, and took it back to my room. That year, my roommate was a person who had lived in many countries most of her life. She was interested, too. There was only one catch - we needed to be fluent in German. Neither of us spoke German, but we decided we could learn it by June - it was March! We studied every night. Our parents signed the work contracts. We left for Germany in June.

Through June and July, we worked in Germany, then toured Norway and Sweden. On our return trip to Germany, we stopped in Copenhagen. On the 'Walking Street,' my roommate recognized a vest a man was wearing. She suspected it was from Asia. She went right up to the person and found out that the vest was from Turkey. The next conversation gave birth to the biggest decision I would make in my young life. To go or not to go on an English double-decker bus to India? I remember sitting down on the steps in the center of Copenhagen so I could think. I would forfeit my plane ticket home and not return for my junior year in college! I asked myself, would this opportunity ever come again? In those few moments I made a decision that changed my entire life. The physical trip went from Turkey to India. The mental trip went from understanding, to tolerance and compassion, and respect for all human beings. The journey continues to remind me that curiosity is a really good quality and can teach so much.

~ *Katie Blum-Katz, M.A., ACE*

Katie Blum-Katz, MA, ACE, Katkoaching, LLC, is a dancer, teacher, trainer, and coach. She founded Katkoaching, LLC, where she coaches individuals and families with ADHD. Katie's MA in Dance Education, ACE certification for exercise, and teaching degree in Theatre, provide a rich background for coaching ADHD clients. Katie is passionate about exercise as partial treatment for ADHD. She has been teaching dance/exercise for 34 years. She began individual coaching in 2000. Ask about her "Tools you can use…"®, via email Katie@katkoaching.com, or www.katkoaching.com. Or just call: 410-757-8830. This is Katie's 3rd time contributing to the ADHD Awareness Book Project

What's Your "Study Style?"

Many people know their "learning style": they are a visual, auditory, kinesthetic or tactile learner. However, knowing your "study style" or where/how/when you do your best work or learning, is equally valuable. To figure out your "study style," ask yourself:

- Do I focus best in a quiet environment or where there is some background noise/activity?
- Do I like everything spread around me or pay attention better in a tidy environment?
- Do I learn best alone or with others?
- When do I do my best? In the morning/afternoon/early evening or night?

The answers to these questions can help you understand how you learn best and know your "study style."

~Laurie Dupar, PMHNP, RN, PCC

Laurie Dupar, PMHNP, RN, PCC is a trained Psychiatric Nurse Practitioner and 12 year veteran ADHD coach specializing in mentoring and training emerging ADHD Coaches.
www.coachingforadhd.com   support@coachingforadhd.com

"You have to find what sparks a light in you so that you in your own way can illuminate the world."

~ Oprah Winfrey

A Red Nose Day

Having ADHD has always been a wonderful gift. I was diagnosed twenty years ago, just after my son was diagnosed. We both have a zest for life that has given us much happiness in the things we do for others and ourselves.

One day we both put on red noses and mapped out a course that our noses could follow. It happened to be senior citizen day at the first store we entered. At first the elderly men and women stared at us with sad faces.

As we smiled and said hello they started to laugh and talk to us.

When we were ready to leave they thanked us for bringing fun and happiness to their lives that day. We really made a difference in the lives of others and you can too. You don't even have to wear a red nose!

~ Barb Rosenfeld

Barb Rosenfeld, founder/past president of ADD of Missouri, is a Healing Touch Practitioner, Reiki Master, retired Special Ed teaching assistant, Professional Clown and Magician.

Self-Efficacy For All Women

L ittle girls receive very different messages from society about their abilities than little boys. Girls are praised for being pretty and obedient. Boys are praised for conquering obstacles. This causes women and men to handle setbacks and stumbling blocks differently.

Unfortunately, these childhood messages convince many women that success and failure are qualities that are part of them and cannot be changed, making it more difficult for women to push through roadblocks.

Society also sends powerful messages to women that they must be perfect, all the time, in every situation. So as women, we try to excel as females, friends, mothers, wives and workers.

But when a woman finds it hard to be perfect, those old messages kick in and she may unconsciously believe she "just doesn't have what it takes." She may blame herself for being imperfect, rather than questioning the reasonableness of society's expectation that she be perfect.

Feeling good about yourself – self-esteem – is wonderful, but a more important quality to develop is self-efficacy. Self-efficacy is knowing that you "can get the job done" in your life. Focusing on pushing through failure even when it's uncomfortable, results in the true self-esteem that comes from being determined to work for and take control of how your life turns out.

Life comes with beauty and majesty, but it also comes with unhappiness and setbacks. Being able to navigate the challenges and obstacles and not labeling them as your "failures" or your "deficiencies" promotes your happiness because you know you have "what it takes to get the job done" even in the face of difficulties.

Above all, recognize that your successes are the result of your efforts, not your innate ability. Praise yourself for tackling problems with a "can do attitude." Redefine "success" as the way you approach a challenge. Acknowledge yourself for any positive step you take in the direction of meeting your goals.

Every night before you go to bed, make it a habit to list at least three things you DID that day to make your life better. In addition to taking responsibility for how your life turns out, remember how important it is to acknowledge yourself for everything you do to move your life forward towards the goals that are meaningful to you. Be aware of just how much your actions influence your life.

~ Dr. Kari Miller, PhD, BCET

Dr. Kari Miller, PhD, ADHD coach and board certified educational therapist, helps women conquer their biggest ADHD challenges. She assists women in getting focused, organized, and motivated so they get unstuck, finish what they start, and accomplish more every day! Dr. Miller leverages her expertise as a learning specialist to help women find unique and exciting strategies for managing their ADHD challenges. Through her group and individual coaching programs and online supportive community, she encourages and inspires women to set their sights high and make big changes in their lives! Visit www.ADHDclearandfocused.com or www.ADHDcoachingforwomen.com Kari.Miller.coach@gmail.com

Special Spot (Keeping Safe)

It can be very hard to keep a preschooler safe and close by you in a busy location like a mall. Suggestion: Make a portable "special spot" from a placemat or hand towel to keep in your purse or vehicle (or several "special spot" mats). This may just be a plain towel or placemat, or you may decorate it with your child. I recommend putting a symbol that your child likes e.g. a star, or teddy bear rather than your child's name. Before using your special spot in public, practice using it at home. Teach your child to stand or sit on his or her special spot. Your child can pretend to be something that stays very still, like a statue or a fawn. I have used this in a parking lot to keep the child in one spot while I turned to close the car door.

~ *Pat Corbett, BEd, MC, MSW*

Pat Corbett (Calgary) is an in-home family support worker at Connections Counseling and Consulting and facilitator at Columbia College. Her dream: bridging gaps. www.reframingthebox.com

Solving Hour-Long Showers

What can they possibly do in there for an hour? And when they emerge some sixty minutes later, with hair still dry and footprints that indicate very little soap was ever used—what's happening?

Think of the bathroom as a time warp! Once in, time ceases to exist when you have ADHD. Bathrooms are the last places in the house most of us consider putting a clock or timer. Without those, how do they know when to emerge from the shower? When the water gets cold, of course!

The solution is simple: stock the bathroom with as many timing devices as you can. Shower clocks for that wash, rinse and repeat cycle. A two-minute liquid timer to make sure teeth are brushed just long enough.

And of course, a wall clock that can be seen from any bathroom position.

~Laurie Dupar, PMHNP, RN, PCC

Laurie Dupar, PMHNP, RN, PCC is a trained Psychiatric Nurse Practitioner and 12 year veteran ADHD coach specializing in mentoring and training emerging ADHD Coaches.
www.coachingforadhd.com support@coachingforadhd.com

"You are amazing.

Remember that."

~Unknown

Need a Vacation?

It's a great feeling to get away on vacation! Whether it includes adventure, relaxation, and/or connection with loved ones, a vacation can be reinvigorating and energizing.

Unfortunately for most of us, vacations don't happen often enough! So, how about creating a mini-vacations for yourself?

Mindful mini-vacations can keep you feeling refreshed and energized. Consider these options:

- Scheduling a weekly candle-lit bath to help focus mindfully on your body sensations.

- Planning a special dessert you anticipate all week, and then eating it slowly and mindfully on Friday night.

- Taking 10 minutes outside daily to listen to the sounds of nature.

- Setting an alarm to ring each afternoon reminding yourself to try a one minute "power pose" to re-energize and focus (see Amy Cuddy's TED Talk at https://www.ted.com/speakers/amy_cuddy).

What type(s) of regular mindful attention might work like a vacation for you?

~ Elizabeth (Liz) Ahmann, ScD, RN, ACC

ADHD Coach, Liz Ahmann, ScD, RN, ACC, also teaches mindfulness classes for individuals with ADHD. Learn more at www.lizahmann.com www.lizahmann.com/mindfulness.html lizahmann.blogspot.com

Wiggle While You Work

Instead of telling students with ADHD to "sit still and get your work done," more teachers are finding success using yoga balls, wiggle seats, and Bouncy Bands to allow students to move while they work.

Cheaper and more durable than yoga balls and wiggle cushions, Bouncy Bands are also constructed with heavy-duty materials. Tired of re-tying therapy bands or inner tubes to desks or chairs? Industrial fasteners keep loops secured on both ends, while support pipes keep the band suspended at the perfect position.

Bouncy Bands attach to student desks and chairs for children (and adults) to bounce their feet and stretch their legs while they work. This sensory relief helps students focus longer, complete more work, stay relaxed during testing, and makes learning more fun than having to sit still for 5-6 hours every day.

~ Scott Ertl, MEd, NBPTS, School Counselor & CEO of Bouncy Bands, LLC

Scott Ertl, school counselor and inventor of Bouncy Bands, promotes active learning to parents and educators to help children learn more effectively. BouncyBands.com

When the Floor is the Biggest Shelf in the Room

Cleaning their room. Organizing is a fight with inevitable chaos when you are a student with ADHD. For whatever reason, the floor becomes the largest shelf in the room...a vertical closet if you will. There, they can spread it out ...where they can see it all...the only problem is this "solution" is a bit like deciding to keep track of the contents of your wallet or purse with your money, credit cards, etc., laid out bare. It makes sense...it just isn't convenient.

As parents, "clean your room" has to be specific. Being clear that all horizontal surfaces must be cleared...including the floor...helps them know exactly what you expect. It may seem silly, but reminding them that "cleaning their room," means that it can't be piled on the floor or their desk or any other horizontal surface, will help them achieve success.

~Laurie Dupar, PMHNP, RN, PCC

Laurie Dupar, PMHNP, RN, PCC is a trained Psychiatric Nurse Practitioner and 12 year veteran ADHD coach specializing in mentoring and training emerging ADHD Coaches.
www.coachingforadhd.com support@coachingforadhd.com

Don't Feed the Trolls

Every ADHD family has one – an Uber-Arguer who can never be out-argued. My client Myra was recounting a recent conversation that resulted when she asked her teenage Uber-Arguer, Michael, to start his homework: "Think about it Mum, if I start my homework now, I'll just do a bad job because I'm tired from concentrating all day at school. It makes more sense for me to play computer games for a while to wind my brain down, and then do my homework. Besides, my coach taught me that I should create bridges for my brain when I am moving from one task to another, and since I will be doing my homework on a computer, my bridge is using a computer game to help my brain transition into homework..."

And before she knew it, she was having a long discussion about bridges, executive functions and the futility of homework. Although she had tried really hard to convince him that his homework needed to be completed before he played computer games, the conversation had ended with her storming off, while he calmly continued to play his game.

In our coaching session Myra came to the realization that such discussions were pointless with her Uber-Arguer. Somehow, after the first 5 seconds of repartee it all became about the argument. The topic was forgotten as he wove a web of words designed to distract her from what he was meant to be doing.

She left our session determined to exercise her newfound wisdom.

A few days later Myra found herself in IKEA with Michael, choosing a cover for the sofa in his bedroom. The colour options were black and grey, and were clearly marked as such on the packaging. She asked him: "Michael what colour would you like? Black or grey?"

"That's not black it's blue. In this light and you can see clearly. How could they possibly call this black? And besides..."

Myra was about to launch into a frustrated tirade about how the item was clearly marked 'black' and why was he being so difficult? But she paused, remembered the promise she had made herself and calmly asked: "Michael what color would you like? Blue or grey?"

To which he conceded with a smile: "You're a wise woman mum, don't feed the trolls. I'll take black."

~ Dr. Michele Toner, PhD, PCC, PCAC

Dr. Michele Toner, PhD, PCC, PCAC, is based in Western Australia, and coaches people from around the world. Her Masters and PhD research, coupled with 20 years of hands-on experience make her well equipped to empower her clients, as they learn to conquer the chaos and stay in control. She works with individuals and their families to identify and harness their strengths, address their challenges, and make ADHD 'work for them.' As a registered mentor coach, Michele also empowers new coaches to be the best they can. www.micheletoner.com

"Sometimes the thoughts in my head get so bored they go out for a stroll through my mouth. This is rarely a good thing."

~ Scott Westerfield

The 3 WACKIEST Things About Having ADHD

1. You don't always think like everyone else... but who cares? Linear thinkers don't always get your wacky way of thinking. You might get lost in the details sometimes, but so what? You're an out-of-the-box thinker who uses creativity to solve problems and brings a fresh perspective to the table!

2. You don't always play it safe... so you have lots of F-U-N! Your ADHD makes you more prone to taking risks, which can definitely make life wacky! That just means you aren't afraid to try something new, like jumping out of a plane! A lot of 'neuro-typical' people would love to have the guts to take risks. Lucky for you, it comes naturally to ADDers!

3. You don't always stick to one thing... but why should you? Your ADHD brain makes you curious about everything. You have lots of interests, meaning you're never bored and can entertain yourself anywhere!

~ *Roya Kravetz, PCC, BCC, CMC, CPE*

Roya Kravetz, Board Certified and Credentialed Coach, specializes in strength-based coaching for individuals whose lives are affected by ADHD and similar Executive Functioning challenges. www.adhdsuccesscoaching.com

Avoiding Something?

Maybe it's counter-intuitive, but often the best way to deal with avoiding something is to find a way to embrace your avoidance.

So instead of thinking you "shouldn't" avoid whatever it is, take some time to pay mindful attention to the avoidance. Here's how:

If you were to welcome the avoidance, what might it be telling you? Notice how you feel about whatever you're avoiding: Overwhelmed? Anxious? Afraid? Confused? Try to examine it non-judgmentally.

Consider writing down what you're avoiding. Become an observer: what stories are you telling yourself about it? What beliefs can you identify? Conversely, what stories and beliefs have you created about avoiding it?

Try extending loving-kindness toward yourself. What might you say to a friend in your shoes? How could you share similar supportive feelings with yourself?

Now ... what's your next step?

~ Elizabeth (Liz) Ahmann, ScD, RN, ACC

ADHD Coach, Liz Ahmann, ScD, RN, ACC, also teaches mindfulness classes for individuals with ADHD. Learn more at www.lizahmann.com www.lizahmann.com/mindfulness.html lizahmann.blogspot.com

My "Brains"

One technique I have found extremely useful to help me keep track of my "to dos" is to print off a copy of my schedule from my online calendar onto an obnoxiously bright colored piece of paper at the beginning of my week. Using this ADD-friendly strategy, I add sticky notes, take handwritten notes from the week on the back, cross off completed tasks, add new or shift "to dos" as they arise during the week. The bright color paper makes it easy to find. At the end of the week, I file it in a drawer in case I need to refer back to it later. As a floor nurse we used a similar system to plan our shift, record and pass on important details and called it our "brains."

~Laurie Dupar, PMHNP, RN, PCC

Laurie Dupar, PMHNP, RN, PCC is a trained Psychiatric Nurse Practitioner and 12 year veteran ADHD coach specializing in mentoring and training emerging ADHD Coaches.
www.coachingforadhd.com support@coachingforadhd.com

Calming the Senses

My husband liked to fish...mainly to walk up and down by the lake and enjoy the sounds of the water lapping at the rocks, watch the silver of the jumping fish, and talk with other fishermen. He rarely brought home a fish, but had a great time. He had a fishing vest covered in pockets. Our son now has that vest. We put little rocks in some of the pockets. You can get rocks at the Dollar Store, but most of the rocks our son has are ones his Dad picked up and polished, making a very special weighted vest. Keeping his hands busy helps our son to keep his attention focused. He will bring along a fidget toy in his pocket - an item that provides stimulation for nerve endings and allows a hands-on/tactile learner to focus. Cat or dollar store toys can make great inexpensive fidget toys.

~ *Pat Corbett, BEd, MC, MSW*

Pat Corbett (Calgary) is an in-home family support worker at Connections Counseling and Consulting and facilitator at Columbia College. Her dream: bridging gaps. www.reframingthebox.com

"My thoughts are like butterflies. They are beautiful, but they fly away."

~ Anonymous

The Power of Empathy

In every one of us is the desire to be heard. One of the most powerful tools in parenting an ADHD child is empathy. We ADHDers know that our emotions can be high intensity, and for our kids, they can lead to maladaptive behaviors because they don't know what to do with those emotions. When a parent acknowledges those intense emotions, it makes a child feel safe. We give them effective outlets for expressing their emotions, but only after we've given them empathy. When our ADHD son feels his high-intensity emotions, we used to fear them, and tried to punish him for feeling them. Now we name them, remind him of his tools to regulate, and those long meltdowns have turned into short waves of emotions.

~ Jared and DeAnn Jennette, Trained Coaches

Jared and DeAnn Jennette are trained life coaches who specialize in families of adopted children with ADHD, SPD, or other "alphabet soup" diagnoses. www.embraceparentcoaching.com embraceparentcoaching@gmail.com

Stories Brought Me Up

Stories got me through life challenges when there was no one else to learn from. It makes me happy to see a growing number of diverse, strong women characters on TV series that I can admire because of their flaws.

I enjoy the ADHD mind of Elsbeth Tascioni, a recurring character on "The Good Wife." Intended as comic relief, Elsbeth portrays the humorous challenges and quirky genius of a deceptively scattered lawyer.

Disapproving glares and eye rolls do not stop her brilliant intellectual maneuvers. She earns the respect of others, even when her mercurial way does not fit the norm of propriety. Although usually too disorganized to premeditate a strategy, she's brilliant and intuitively uses each moment to her advantage. "I don't know how I know half the things I know," she says. Her strength comes from catching her opponents off guard. They don't know what hit them, literally, she's a klutz!

In one scene, she chases a man through a parking lot in heels yelling his name and dropping papers zigzagging between cars. My friend watching the show with me, grinned and said, "I've seen you do that." I was honored!

Her perceived erratic behavior (that ADHDers would see as normal) sometimes gets her into trouble and once got her arrested for assault! Fearful of Elsbeth's propensity to ramble and blurt out an unrelated chain of thoughts, her lawyer advises, "Answer just what you're asked. Then be silent." Good advice from her lawyer, Alicia, who was hoping she would pass a psych evaluation required before posting bail. She didn't make it. She started giggling about the questions, freaked out, and lost her composure.

I love Elsbeth's validating magical flaws and the very particular way she is able to see the world. Like me, numbers she sees sometimes rearrange themselves. Scattered words compose a message and give the precise clue she needs. It is as if the universe is winking at her saying, "You're on the right track!"

She is gifted with noticing beauty and excellence everywhere, making her cheerful and in awe about life. She is loud and colorful with bright red hair, laser-focused in a fight for what is right. But when someone stomps on her boundaries or emotions, she is valiant and does not hesitate in holding them accountable.

"I'm feeling a bit vulnerable, but I'm going to use it." – Elsbeth Tascioni

Brava!

~ *Angelis Iglesias* HSP HSS ADHD Coach Consultant Researcher

Angelis Iglesias, HSP, ADHD Coach, Researcher. I help professionals and business owners develop and expand their business, achieve environmental and emotional regulation, to enjoy satisfying work and relationships. I support Highly Sensitive People with group coaching and research. When the signature core transformation you provide isn't clear and at the forefront, those that really need and want it, can't find you. Build a powerful social media presence. Technology and Social Media Training and Consulting for Coaches in English and Spanish Faculty at Impact Coaching Academy, Ontario, Canada. www.angelisiglesias.com www.mindheartinstitute.com ai@angelisiglesias.com

What is Your Rainbow Playlist?

I learned about a "Rainbow List" from one of my mentors, David Giwerc, owner and director of the ADD Coach Academy. We can make a rainbow list by reflecting on, and writing down, great moments in our lives. It is the kind of list that helps us remember our successes rather than our failures. It's a list we can turn to when we are having a bad day or feeling extra doubtful. We can use it to look back, review, and be reminded of our successes and strengths.

A fun twist on the "Rainbow List" is to create a "Rainbow Playlist" of your favorite or most meaningful songs: a collection of music that will remind you of your strengths to encourage and uplift you.

What would you want on your "Rainbow Playlist?"

~Laurie Dupar, PMHNP, RN, PCC

Laurie Dupar, PMHNP, RN, PCC is a trained Psychiatric Nurse Practitioner and 12 year veteran ADHD coach specializing in mentoring and training emerging ADHD Coaches.
www.coachingforadhd.com support@coachingforadhd.com

Handling Stress: Mine!

Anxiety seems to breed anxiety. The more stressed I became with rooms not being cleaned, children not seeming to listen, not being able to keep a routine well myself...the more anxious the boys became. The more anxious they became, the more they would shut down. They would find something to do that calmed them (often a device such as the TV or computer), which in turn distracted them from the task Mom was ranting about. I was working against myself and against home being a calm and relaxing place. After all, they had to work hard to meet expectations and handle stimulation at school or programs every weekday. Home was a place where they did not have to sit still. I learned to pull out a storybook, or put on a 'family movie,' so we could just enjoy each other and then tackle the tasks.

~ *Pat Corbett, BEd, MC, MSW*

Pat Corbett (Calgary) is an in-home family support worker at Connections Counseling and Consulting and facilitator at Columbia College. Her dream: bridging gaps. www.reframingthebox.com

"Taken together, it's almost a sure sign. The letters float off the page when you read, right? That's because your mind is hardwired for ancient Greek. And the ADHD-you're impulsive, can't sit still in the classroom. That's your battlefield reflex. In a real fight, they'd keep you alive. As for the attention problems, that's because you see too much, Percy, not too little. Your senses are better than a regular mortal's."

~ Rick Riordan, The Lightning Thief

Five Communication Secrets That Can Change Your ADHD Relationship Forever

Got ADHD relationship communication "challenges?" Here are five top tips that can save your marriage/partnership/love life:

Secret #1: Say "Ouch!" Early and Often. Resentment builds quickly when either one of you withholds your true feelings.

Secret #2: Speak Your Truth and Only Your Truth. Take a moment to check in with yourself to identify your true feelings, then begin the conversation.

Secret #3: Ask Clarifying Questions. Instead of arguing your position, have an inquiring mind to get more information about your partner's position. Ask "Could you say more about that?"

Secret # 4: Ask for What You Want. Your partner is not a mind reader. You have to articulate what you want. Ask, ask, ask, ask, ask, ask, ASK.

Secret # 5: Know When to Hold 'Em. Timing is everything; set an appointment to talk instead of diving in when emotions run high. Simple, but not easy. Keep practicing!

~ Linda Roggli, PCC

Linda Roggli, PCC, helps stop the madness for midlife ADHD women through startlingly effective coaching, transformational retreats and weekend intensives. You ready? http://addiva.net http://addivaretreats.com linda@addiva.net

Surprise! Wake up Brain!

Try this strategy when you need to focus for long periods or concentrate deeply, such as comprehending difficult reading material or paying close attention to details. This strategy relies on your brain's tendency to "revive" through novelty and surprise.

First, gather together pictures and items that appeal to you. The following "surprise gifts" work particularly well – pictures of your spouse or child, objects that symbolize success in your life, words or sayings that motivate you to excel, pictures of favorite vacation spots, photos that capture meaningful experiences in your life.

The second step is to "hide" these inspirational objects in "random" places, for example in the book you are reading, in the desk drawers, or underneath something you use during the task. As you "come upon" these jewels of pleasurable inspiration while completing the task, you'll receive a boost in brain stimulation, energy and focus!

~ Dr. Kari Miller, PhD, BCET

Dr. Kari Miller, ADHD coach and educational therapist, helps women focus and organize so they get more done and finish what they start! www.ADHDclearandfocused.com Kari.Miller.coach@gmail.com

Beat the Blues

Some of my favorite coaching clients are students. I love working with them as they discover more successful ways to manage their academic challenges. One of these strategies is simply to get them to use a planner. They start out the school year very enthusiastic, but often by winter break they are "bored." They stop entering due dates and start missing homework assignments. At the start of winter term, in order to restart their interest in a once-successful strategy, I present them with a "beat the winter blues" student kit. The new highlighters, pens and sticky notes for their planner renew their interest and have them back on track for success.

~Laurie Dupar, PMHNP, RN, PCC

Laurie Dupar, PMHNP, RN, PCC is a trained Psychiatric Nurse Practitioner and 12 year veteran ADHD coach specializing in mentoring and training emerging ADHD Coaches.
www.coachingforadhd.com   support@coachingforadhd.com

Make a Micro-Change

"That note worked for a couple of weeks, and then I started ignoring it."

"I really liked that planner, but after a while I just stopped using it."

"I set a reminder in my phone, but I don't even hear it anymore."

Folks with ADHD need external cues and systems to help them to follow through. But often, after developing an effective strategy and putting it in place, the strategy seems to fade.

The ADHD mind craves the new and surprising. So instead of throwing your strategy out the window, try a micro-change.

Examples of micro-changes:

• Using a different color pen or paper,

• Moving your clock to a new location,

• Changing a ring tone or app for an alarm,

• Rearranging your desk at work.

To develop your own micro-changes, ask: What is the smallest possible change I can make so my strategy feels new again?

~ Casey Dixon, SCAC, BCC, MSEd

Casey Dixon is Success Strategist and ADHD Coach employing a
unique focus on science-based, innovative strategies for demand-
ridden professionals with ADHD. www.mindfullyadd.com
www.dixonlifecoaching.com,

"Behold the turtle:

He only makes progress

when he sticks his neck out."

~ James Bryant Conant

Find Your Zen Where You Can

L iving with ADHD is an exercise in living with paradox. Some of my ADHD gifts are an intense curiosity, enthusiasm for life and learning new things. This tendency towards "YES!" can also lead me to overwhelm and spinning my wheels. Not knowing where to start with the many activities on my plate can get in the way of participating in life in ways I would like.

Before a later-in-life diagnosis, my go-to strategy for getting things done was to push through, work harder and longer. There came a point when that was no longer a reliable option. I've been on quite a learning curve, becoming more aware of strategies that work or don't work for me and experimenting with creating new healthier habits. I have enjoyed benefits from various practices such as mindfulness, yoga, Qi Gong, meditation, and deep breathing, and know their value. When overwhelm hits though, these are often the first to go as I spin off into frustration and indecision.

One particular morning, facing a longer than usual to-do list, deadlines looming, with a lack of sleep as a backdrop, a day of overwhelm and inertia was threatening on the horizon. It was a proud moment when I caught myself, pulled back and deliberately chose NOT to go there. I remembered seeing an online meditation to address overwhelm, decided to start there and hopefully proceed through my day with clarity. As I tried to switch the all-in-one computer/television/satellite system from TV viewing to computer use, a crash 'em up movie blared through the speakers, adding to my frustration as I fumbled, fussed and cursed in vain. Any momentary hope I'd had for proceeding with calm and clarity vanished.

I stepped back from the tangle of wires to see Terminator 3 playing: a crazy chase scene full of destruction and mayhem. It was so ridiculously funny, and surprisingly, watching big things get blown up and wiped out by an angry female cyborg driving a wide load construction vehicle bent on destroying Arnold Schwarzenegger's character was incredibly cathartic. That 10-minute scene was as good as a 10-minute meditation! I felt much lighter and ready to tackle the to-do list.

Even the tools in my toolbox are paradoxical, but I'm glad to have discovered choices to deal with overwhelm ranging from accessing a calm center through meditation to channeling my inner cyborg in a single-minded pursuit of a goal.

~ Anne Marie Nantais, OCT, AAC

Anne Marie Nantais is an ADHD coach (AAC) and an Ontario Certified Teacher (OCT) with 19 years of classroom and Special Education experience. She started "ADHD and Beyond: Coaching, Tutoring, and Consulting Services" to help people of all ages go beyond the label of ADHD and into living their best lives. With compassion and deep listening, she works with clients to help them find personalized, unique solutions using their strengths to create the energy and ease they crave in their lives. Anne Marie connects with her clients over phone, Skype, or in-person.

www.adhdandbeyond.com   amn8@mnsi.net (519)735-1177

Why Did I Come into this Room?

Okay, I do this a lot. Forgetting why I'm walking into this room or another in the house. As I walk, "to do" items come into my thoughts and throw off my concentration. This can wreak havoc for an ADHD brain. My suggestion is this: find a spot or an object in each room in your house that is your memory trigger. When you look in that direction it tells your brain that you are ready to get that information back. The thought is still there, it just got pushed back for a moment. Take a deep breath, and trust that your memory trigger will bring it back. The more you allow yourself to relax in the moment, the more likely the information will "pop back." Pressure shuts down our brain. Give it a shot!

~ Silvia Razon, ADHD Coach

Silvia Razon, ADHD Coach at Focused Intentions ADHD Coaching, partners with all ages in navigating ADHD life.
www.focusedadhdcoach.com   support@focusedadhdcoach.com
(650) 235 - 9344

Time Outs are Not Just for Toddlers

In our family of four children, two with ADHD, emotional impulsivity ran high. Playfulness could quickly turn from overwhelm to anger—not just for my kids, but for me, too..

One day my son, age 8, took friends on a tour of our new home. Passing the laundry room, he explained, "This is where Mom takes her time-outs." For clarification, his friends asked, "This is where you take your time-outs?" "No," he replied, "this is where *Mom* takes her time-outs."

The laundry room was a sanctuary for me when things got overwhelming and I wanted to avoid getting out of control. Behind closed doors I would breathe deeply until my emotions settled.

When your emotions threaten to erupt, give yourself permission to take a time-out, get back in control, and be the sane adult and parent your children need.

~Laurie Dupar, PMHNP, RN, PCC

Laurie Dupar, PMHNP, RN, PCC is a trained Psychiatric Nurse Practitioner and 12 year veteran ADHD coach specializing in mentoring and training emerging ADHD Coaches. www.coachingforadhd.com support@coachingforadhd.com

Desktop Dopamine Dosers

Hate to file? Avoid paying bills? Try this simple tip to get your brain chemistry on your side, working for you, not against you!

Brain chemicals called neurotransmitters play a key role in helping us tackle those "boring" and "nasty" tasks. One of these neurotransmitters is dopamine – the major chemical that regulates focus, movement and pleasurable feelings.

Try some of these dopamine dosers to get your brain ready to tackle "tedious" desktop chores such as filing, bill paying, and report writing.

Set out objects in your workspace that are attractive or have personal meaning for you – such as pictures of your family, colorful containers and pens, and snow globes. Wear your favorite color clothing or jewelry or wear something that is special to you in some way.

Be sure to look at your "dopamine dosers" frequently throughout the day to help you stay happy and focused!

~ *Dr. Kari Miller, PhD, BCET*

Dr. Kari Miller, ADHD coach and educational therapist, helps women focus and organize so they get more done and finish what they start! www.ADHDclearandfocused.com Kari.Miller.coach@gmail.com

"Always be a first-rate version of yourself, instead of a second-rate version of somebody else."

~ Judy Garland

Don't Hit Yourself on the Way Down!

Lying still is sooooo boring that it can make it harder to fall asleep, so try one of these whacky ways to get you passed the boredom so you can get to the land of nod. If you're tired, but having trouble falling asleep, try holding your arm up in the air as though you want to be called on in class. You'd be surprised both by how many people do this and how well it works for them--and somehow no one ever hits themselves when their hand comes down! You can also try moving your toes back and forth against the sheets. Or fiddling with a bit of blanket or a button on your PJs. You'd be surprised how well these strategies work!

~ Sarah D. Wright

Sarah D. Wright works with clients to help them become more effective and get them back on track. Contact her at Sarah@SarahDWright.com

Put on Your War Glitter

We've all had them. Those days when we can't seem to muster up motivation from anywhere let alone finish an important project, etc. One of the most creative solutions came from a student of mine who solved this dilemma by putting on her war glitter.

What's war glitter and how do you put it on? Well, it seems the best way to put on your war glitter is to start with a tube of clear lip balm. Draw a half circle about an inch under your eyes with the lip balm (any flavor will do) imitating the eye black half circles seen on athletes to minimize the glare of the lights and sun. Next, gently apply eye makeup friendly glitter over the lip balm, brushing off any excess, to get that fun and wacky, "ready to rumble" attitude!

~Laurie Dupar, PMHNP, RN, PCC

Laurie Dupar, PMHNP, RN, PCC is a trained Psychiatric Nurse Practitioner and 12 year veteran ADHD coach specializing in mentoring and training emerging ADHD Coaches.
www.coachingforadhd.com support@coachingforadhd.com

The Shadow Game

A favorite game when my husband and I went for a walk with our sons was the Shadow Game. This worked best for us when the shadow was in front of me. The object was for the child to stay in the parent's shadow as we walked along the sidewalk. Sometimes we would add special directions like "shuffle your feet for the next 3 squares," "hop for 2 squares," "sneak 3 squares, stop until [Mom] catches up and steal a hug," and so on. If we were getting close to a crossing, I would call "freeze" for them to stand still until I caught up to hold their hands. Sometimes, Mom had to stay in the child's shadow. This would keep the boys on the sidewalk, close to me while giving them lots of movement and fun.

~ *Pat Corbett, BEd, MC, MSW*

Pat Corbett (Calgary) is an in-home family support worker at Connections Counseling and Consulting and facilitator at Columbia College. Her dream: bridging gaps. www.reframingthebox.com

Do You Want to Be Right or Happy?

Do you find yourself constantly battling with your kids or even other adults? It's important to defend your perspective, but constant arguing can damage relationships. Too often, no one wins.

Arguments are usually all about opinion, and there is no way to prove who is "right." But once our ego gets attached to a point of view, it's hard to recognize when we've reached a stalemate.

That makes it all the more important to pick our battles with loved ones. Sometimes, that means letting go of the need to prove a point.

So, next time you find yourself in one of these situations, hoping to convince someone that you are right, try asking yourself, "Would I rather be right? Or is this a good time to let it go, and choose to be happy, instead?"

~Diane Dempster & Elaine Taylor-Klaus, Co-Founders, ImpactADHD.com

Diane Dempster, MHSA, PCC, CPC and Elaine Taylor-Klaus, PCC, CPCC, the parenting coaches of ImpactADHD.com, the leading online resource for parents of kids with ADHD.

"And wouldn't we be better off
if every New Year's,
we thought about the things we did
right and we resolved to keep doing
them, no matter how wacky they
were."

~ Lisa Scottoline

The Monster Binder

When I was in middle school, I had one of those ubiquitous 3-ring binders, called a "loose-leaf," made of stylish blue jean material. This was the required storage system to hold class work from every class, neatly separated by colored tabs. However, this system didn't work out well for me. First of all, some of the teachers didn't hole-punch their papers, so I didn't know where to place them. Secondly, those that were hole-punched occasionally got ripped and fell out. Finally, whenever I accidentally dropped the binder on the floor, the bindings would un-bind, and all the papers would fall all over the place. Needless to say, this binder system did not keep me organized.

In high school, I vowed to never use another 3-ring binder, so I bought a small spiral notebook with an attached folder for each class. This was much more manageable and worked fine for me.

Fast forward to adulthood and helping my own children be organized. When my daughter Emily was in 6th grade, the teachers required one large binder for all subjects to keep the students organized. Luckily, the binders had improved since my day. They were shiny and came in different colors, and inside you can fit a 3-hole puncher and pencil case. Best of all,

Emily's binder wrapped around itself to prevent its contents from spilling. The rings were built better, too, and stayed shut. The problem was that as the year rolled on, the binder became bigger and bigger until it took on a life of its own. We tried to take out papers that were no longer needed, but just the same, it kept growing. This became very overwhelming for Emily, who, to keep things more manageable, started taking out some of the binder's contents. Finally, one day she came home and announced that the binder was lost. I asked her how such a large binder could be lost, but she said it just was. We looked everywhere in our house, and then I came to her school. We searched every one of her classes, including each desk, the cafeteria, and the "lost and found." We never found it. At the end of the exhaustive search, she admitted to me that she had already taken out everything she needed, so nothing important was in there anyway.

When Emily started high school, we purchased a few binders and folders. As time went on, we modified the system. Some subjects had so much material that each required its own binder, while other subjects could share a binder. Many teachers do not hole-punch, and Emily couldn't find the time to punch holes herself, so she used her folders – a lot – until they became huge. When this happened, we took out the old papers from the bottom and got a new folder for the remaining papers. This folder system would drive some people crazy but worked well for Emily. And although she has block scheduling, she takes everything with her and travels around with her backpack all day to avoid misplacing anything. Her back is strong and she keeps track of everything most of the time.

My other daughter, Bethany, started out with mostly binders and now has folders, which she switches every morning, depending on the day's classes. She manages to keep track and have the right materials on the right days.

It is important for students to find personal organization systems that work for them. Parents, tutors, and coaches can help. It may take some time, but it is worth the effort. Don't get stuck with a monster binder!

~ Cheryl Feuer Gedzelman

Cheryl Feuer Gedzelman is President of Tutoring For Success, located in the Washington, DC area, which provides home based tutoring, SAT/ACT and SSAT test prep, and academic coaching in the Washington DC metro area. Cheryl has helped children with diverse needs succeed since 1994. She personally interviews highly qualified tutors and offers consulting to clients.
www.TutoringForSuccess.com (703) 390-9220

Are You Jet Lagged?

Every weekend, people with ADHD are living a jet set lifestyle, flying from one coast and back again in a couple of days. Not literally, but when you stay up late or sleep in late, your body reacts to this like jet lag.

Sleeping with ADHD is already challenging. Every time you alter your sleep, or waking time more than an hour, it takes your body and brain three days to recover. So, when you stay up late on Friday or sleep until noon on Saturday, it takes your body and ADHD brain until Wednesday to readjust.

Going to bed and getting up at the same time, consistently, is one of the most effective strategies to managing your ADHD symptoms. So keep those sleep times regular, or you will feel like you jetted around the globe without enjoying the scenery.

~Laurie Dupar, PMHNP, RN, PCC

Laurie Dupar, PMHNP, RN, PCC is a trained Psychiatric Nurse Practitioner and 12 year veteran ADHD coach specializing in mentoring and training emerging ADHD Coaches.
www.coachingforadhd.com support@coachingforadhd.com

I Know I Put it Someplace!

You have a special, important thing you don't want to misplace – a passport, favorite jewelry or the speech you wrote for your daughter's wedding. You put the "important thing" away in a special place where it won't get lost, where you know it will be safe.

And then you forget where that special place is.

Here is my advice to avoid this heartbreaking scenario: Write the whereabouts of your special item on a card, then place the card where it will be seen at the right time. For example, put one in your suitcase that reads "PASSPORT IS IN ZIPPERED POCKET OF THIS SUITCASE." Then put another one in your trip file – you aren't limited to one card!

Next time you ask, "Has anyone seen the speech I wrote?" You may hear "Dad, look in the pocket of your suit. That's what the card on the fridge says!

~ Steven Freedman, MA, MBA, ADHD Coach

Steven Freedman, MA, MBA, ADHD Coach and Support Group facilitator, helps adults with ADHD get things done.
www.ADHDCoachingForResults.com
Steven@ADHDCoachingForResults.com (443)310-1392

Don't Worry, Your Child Will Get Distracted. Or You Will.

Almost every ADHD child has an ADHD parent. And we ADHD parents can come up with great parenting plans. The problem is if they don't work immediately, or something disrupts our plan, the plan is forgotten. Just as our kids get distracted from what we've asked (no matter how many times we've asked), so will we. And often when we get distracted, we feel overwhelmed and insecure as a parent. We put too much pressure on ourselves, and our kids feel that. Perfectly executing our plans isn't the goal: creating a safe space for your child to grow is. So don't sweat their distraction. When you recognize it, take a breath, remind yourself of the goal, and get back to it. The good news is, you'll forget about it soon enough.

~ Jared and DeAnn Jennette

Jared and DeAnn Jennette are trained coaches who specialize in families of adopted children with ADHD, SPD and other "alphabet soup" diagnoses. www.embraceparentcoaching.com embraceparentcoaching@gmail.com

"He who laughs...lasts."

~ Erma Bombeck

Create an Action Board!

An "action board" is a tool that can help you focus on what is important to you.

It's a vision board with pictures, words, quotations, and items that catch your eye or inspire you. NO SHOULDS! If a picture grabs your attention, looks or feels right, tear it out! If you have goals in mind, grab pictures of action steps as well. Then paste your collection onto a big piece of paper and look at what goal or goals the board inspires. Finally, title it, identify steps, and consider target dates toward your goal(s).

In the process of creating an action board, we spend time considering our goal(s), finding the right pictures, and putting them together. We literally *see*: "This is important" and "This is how to achieve it." This clarity and motivation can propel us to action!

~Laurie Dupar, PMHNP, RN, PCC

Laurie Dupar, PMHNP, RN, PCC is a trained Psychiatric Nurse Practitioner and 12 year veteran ADHD coach specializing in mentoring and training emerging ADHD Coaches.
www.coachingforadhd.com support@coachingforadhd.com

Forget Me Not

Losing and forgetting things can be so frustrating! To keep this from happening, try these out-of-the-box ideas:

Make it colorful! Put your keys on a bright keychain or lanyard. Use the brightest dry erase markers on whiteboards to catch your attention. Cover your phone in a bright phone case or maybe even a glow in the dark one to find them easily. Carry a bright colored wallet or purse so you can spot it anywhere in the room!

Hang it! Use hooks, or basket with hooks, to hang those important items. Hang keys on a designated hook by the door. Capture thoughts by hanging whiteboards in every room or on the back of every door of the house.

Make it a habit! Park your car in the same spot at shopping centers, malls or events. Take a picture of what you want to remember to add to your planner later.

~ Stephanie J. Noel Kirlin, ADHD Coach

Stephanie J. Noel Kirlin, Executive, Leadership, Life and ADHD Coach in Santa Barbara, CA. Helps clients find clarity,fun and achieve personal success. www.bridgingyourworldstogether.com Stephanie@bridgingyourworldstogether.com

ADHD and Rockin' It!

I love live music, and I would love to be in a rock band. When I was younger I rocked out in front of the mirror. So I'm learning to play the keyboard. How do I get myself to practice, which is one of the hardest things for an ADHDer to do? When I go to concerts, I take videos. I imagine myself on stage performing on stage.

When I get home I watch those recordings and remember the excitement I felt in that moment. With my calendar, I map out the daily times I'm going to practice. Then I set my icalendar to alert me with a favorite song at practice times. When I hear Madonna, it's time to jam! I play the video to get myself in that musical mood, so I can tap into that enthusiasm from the concert. Then I start jamming on the piano!

~ Candace Sahm, MA Ed, JST Coach Training

Candace Sahm, MA Ed, ADHD Coach and Special Educator with JST Coach training. Supports youth and adults to reach their highest potential. 25 years experience.

Making a Focus Bubble

As children, our sons shared a bedroom. When bedtime routine was done both would fidget and move about in bed. To settle them, I would do a 'magic trick' where I would sit on the floor between their beds, close my eyes, and breathe deeply. They would "match" my rate of breathing and fall sleep.

Our most productive or focused talks have been in the car with no TV to distract or place to wander off to. We shut out extra sounds (keep the radio or music off while we talk). Our son once said while we sat in a traffic jam, "Oh good! More quality time to chat." For long-distance drives, we collected audio books. Even when they were very little, we used Star Trek or Star Wars novels, which would last almost the whole trip. They enjoyed hearing the stories repeatedly and we seldom heard "are we almost there?"

~ *Pat Corbett, BEd, MC, MSW*

Pat Corbett (Calgary) is an in-home family support worker at Connections Counseling and Consulting and facilitator at Columbia College. Her dream: bridging gaps. www.reframingthebox.com

Is Your "Filter" Full?

Having ADHD means that the brain is busy most of the time with an assortment of thoughts or ideas. Having ADHD also means that we are less likely to have the full ability to filter our thoughts or stimuli in the environment. If we are not taking the time each day to check and see if our 'filter is full,' this hyperactivity or overabundance of mental or environmental activity can often lead to feeling overwhelmed and eventually shutting down. It's a bit like the difference between experiencing the world with gentle waves washing up on the beach, verses a tsunami that completely washes us out! Making sure we are pausing during our day to clear our thoughts, or download them into a planner or other reminder system, will help to keep that filter clear so we can move forward.

~Laurie Dupar, PMHNP, RN, PCC

Laurie Dupar, PMHNP, RN, PCC is a trained Psychiatric Nurse Practitioner and 12 year veteran ADHD coach specializing in

mentoring and training emerging ADHD Coaches.
www.coachingforadhd.com support@coachingforadhd.com

Your Seven (Yes, Seven!) Senses

When your busy mind needs grounding, try sensory integration (SI) strategies to get back in your body and stay on task. SI is how your brain interprets, integrates sensory stimulation. Identify your preferences to awaken/calm your 7 senses!

Visual (From clothing to couch): Inattentive? Add bright colors, simple décor!

Hyperactive? Try soft colors; decrease busy patterns; declutter!

Overwhelmed? Enlist TaskRabbit.com (for one-off tasks), friends, or a professional organizer

Olfactory: Scented candles; essential oils on a handkerchief/scarf

Alerting: citrus, peppermint. Relaxing: vanilla, lavender

Auditory: Music; guided meditation; sound apps (e.g. ocean waves, white noise)

Touch: Cook; paint; draw; knit; fidgets of varying size, pliability, material

Taste: Sour/peppermint candy; fresh fruit

Proprioceptive (How your body feels in space): Push, pull, carry, lift heavy stuff

Heavy backpack/briefcase on your lap

Weighted: vest, blanket, lap pad* (like your dentist's!)

Form-fitting clothing, Chin-ups

Vestibular (balance, movement): Rocking chair; swing; inverted yoga poses

Sense to soar!

~ Ariel Davis, ADHD Coach

Ariel Davis, ADHD Coach/Occupational Therapy Master's Candidate, uses her experience with dual-diagnosed teens/adults and the

crea____ ____iscover and build client strengths.
www ____ gthscoach.com ADHDstrengthscoach@gmail.com

Please Don't Make Me Adult

Since childhood, I've experienced "slowness" being a strength. Contrary to my most natural ability to lose track of time passing, my ultimate adult challenge lies in giving up the perceived control over time, which drives my thinly stretched planning powers.

Often my body protests against busyness (the illusionary need to prove myself through performance!) that plays out in

- Overbooked schedules

- Inadequate daily replenishment

- "As-soon-as" survival thinking

- Debilitating overwhelm.

From daily schedule planning attempts, I've clarified:

- Allocating ENOUGH TIME = NO RUSHING NEEDED whatsoever

- FORCED changes do NOT work well.

Unexpectedly, a way to rather LOVE THE NEEDED CHANGES INTO BEING, was paved along with a WhatsApp image of a dog authentically stating "I can't adult today...please don't make me adult."

These words struck home! Magically, they help realign my mind, heart and body as they are becoming manifested in scheduled "JUST BE" time!

~ Sanlia Marais PACG,CC

Sanlia Marais, professional ADHD/Consciousness Coach, supports clients towards empowered relationships via radical self-care and

appreciation for their emotions and innate strengths.
www.entreecreativechange.com   sanlia@entreecreativechange.com

Pause to Ponder Positively

Does negative thinking or worry take up too much time in your ADHD thinking? If so, it is time to take back your brain with *positive* thinking.

Positive thinking means approaching life's challenges with a positive outlook. It does not mean avoiding or ignoring the bad things; instead, it involves making the most of potentially bad situations, trying to see the best in other people, and viewing yourself and your abilities in a positive light.

Try these:

1. Become aware of negative thinking and notice when it happens.
2. Be willing to give equal time to positive thoughts like what went well, what you learned and what's possible to do differently.
3. Repeat 1 and 2!

Positive thinking helps you tackle life's challenges by focusing on your strengths and growth, as well as tuning in to effective solutions to problems.

~Laurie Dupar, PMHNP, RN, PCC

Laurie Dupar, PMHNP, RN, PCC specializes in mentoring and training emerging ADHD Coaches. www.coachingforadhd.com support@coachingforadhd.com

"I was trying to daydream but my mind kept wandering."

~ Steven Wright

Mind Mapping in Reverse

One of my clients had difficulty with the monotony of to-do lists. She was a visual processor, even an amateur sketch artist, so we talked about using mind mapping as a visual way to break big tasks into manageable ones. That worked well for a time, but then she hit a wall.

It became difficult for her to recognize her successes when she got sidetracked and 'life happened' to derail her mind mapped plan.

A new idea occurred to her: a reverse mind map! At the end of each day she drew a map of what she had actually done that day, especially those things that happened that weren't planned.

She realized by using this tool that she really did accomplish a lot. She was even able to acknowledge her successes. Since then her progress with the 'normal' mind map and the 'reverse' mind map has been truly amazing!

~ Valerie C Krupp

Valerie Krupp, BMEd, MALS, is an ADHD Coach who helps adult clients put the puzzle pieces of ADHD together to create their best life. Visit her at ADDultLifeCoaching.com (803) 413-7398

Don't Teach Kids to Lie (or How to Teach Kids NOT To Lie)

All kids lie sometimes. We hear it a lot. "My son said he'd done his homework." "My daughter said she didn't go to her friends." "He lied to me." "She looked right at me and lied."

ADHD kids, especially, are given to "Defensive Denial," and we parents are partially to blame. We correct them all day, with constant re-directions. And they get tired of being wrong.

So they come up with ways to be right. Can you blame them? Imagine feeling "wrong" all the time! What's a parent to do?

• Take the shame, blame, annoyance and embarrassment out of your corrections, and make them "matter of fact."

• Limit corrections– do you need to correct every bad table manner at every meal?

• When you correct a behavior, make sure you do it without anything in your voice that makes them feel "bad" or "wrong" for a simple mistake.

~ Diane Dempster & Elaine Taylor-Klaus, Co-Founders, ImpactADHD.com

Diane Dempster, MHSA, PCC, CPC and Elaine Taylor-Klaus, PCC, CPCC, the parenting coaches of ImpactADHD.com, the leading online resource for parents of kids with ADHD.

Keeping Focused (Textbooks)

When our son was in grade 4, a new math text was introduced with lots of pictures, color and action on each page. His teacher recognized that when she asked him to read the math question, he could not find it...a consistent pattern across several pages. She tried an older book that had mainly math questions and facts with some simple line drawings in black and white. He was able to locate the question and work to figure it out. She requested and received permission to use the older book where our son could identify where to place his focus. The text that used many pictures and colors was over stimulating for him and the question or fact, which should be the focus, did not stand out for him. Thank goodness for educators like this one (detectives and problem solvers). Yay Educators and Advocates!

~ Pat Corbett, BEd, MC, MSW

Pat Corbett (Calgary) is an in-home family support worker at Connections Counseling and Consulting and facilitator at Columbia College. Her dream: bridging gaps. www.reframingthebox.com

Scribbles, Scrawls and Solutions (To Truly Horrible Handwriting)

When I travel and send postcards back to friends, they tell me the cards take on new meaning each time they read them because my truly illegible handwriting is so difficult to decipher!

The solution? Technology.

Now I compose my postcard message on my laptop or phone, take a quick photo of the postcard, attach it to my text message and voila! My "having a great time, wish you were here" greetings arrive intact (and faster, although without the cool foreign stamps).

I use my beloved Brother labeler to keep my files accessible (translate: legible) to my assistant, but I also label leftovers in the fridge, light switches and my earring drawer.

For true hands-off writing, I turn to the built-in voice activated assistant in my phone. Not always 100% accurate, but at least the printing is legible. And my friends are happy again.

~ *Linda Roggli, PCC*

Linda Roggli, PCC, helps stop the madness for midlife ADHD women through startlingly effective coaching, transformational retreats and weekend intensives. You ready? addiva.net addivaretreats.com linda@addiva.net

An ADHD Conundrum

Why are stimulants used when someone is hyperactive? This is one of ADHD's biggest brainteasers! You see, the physical hyperactivity seen in some people with ADHD is actually a symptom of inactivity of the brain. When people are moving about, restless, the physical movement of the body helps to increase the amount of dopamine available to the brain.

Not enough dopamine getting to the front part of the brain is the main problem thought to cause ADHD. Without full access to this part of the brain responsible for executive function, the ability to pay attention, focus on things less interesting, stop before we act, etc., is nearly impossible. It's a bit like expecting someone with a vision problem to simply "focus" so that they can see better; not happening!

~Laurie Dupar, PMHNP, RN, PCC

Laurie Dupar, PMHNP, RN, PCC is a trained Psychiatric Nurse Practitioner and 12 year veteran ADHD coach specializing in mentoring and training emerging ADHD Coaches. www.coachingforadhd.com   support@coachingforadhd.com

From Our Family to Yours

Pat Corbett (BEd, MC, MSW), Calgary, Alberta, dedicates this submission to her husband, Len Corbett (diagnosed in his 50's), and their sons, two young men with an alphabet soup of challenges including ADHD and ASD.

Len was a man rich in curiosity, loved to learn, and was most settled when walking in the woods or near a river. His sons meant the world to him. Pat cherishes the words of her eldest son: "My guardian angel is heaving a sigh of relief and throwing a party, because Dad is there to take over."

Pat works in the in-home program at an agency that systemically supports families where a parent has an intellectual impairment and as an adjunct facilitator in the Human Services program at Columbia College. Her dream is to help lessen the gaps and build on strengths for individuals and workers in the field.

~ *Patricia (Pat) Corbett, BEd, MC, MSW*

Pat Corbett, mother, family member and ally hopes to partner with her son to develop photo books to help bridge gaps for individuals and workers. Her new website is called www.reframingthebox.com

Tom Sawyer Knew a Thing or Two

The character, Tom Sawyer can teach us a thing or two about getting things done. Remember the story about whitewashing the fence? He made it seem like such fun that he got the other kids to do his chore for him! There are two lessons here. One is to turn chores into a game: see how much you can get done in a small period of time, or better yet, race someone to see who can get the most done in that short period of time! The other is delegate! Particularly for women, delegating seems to be hard, but if you can get someone else to do that task, you'll be able to get that much more done. Tom was a slick talker, but I bet with your creative ADHD brain you can figure out how to make a task more entertaining, for yourself and for others.

~ Sarah D. Wright

Sarah D. Wright works with clients to help them become more effective and get them back on track. Contact her at Sarah@SarahDWright.com

Just Laugh...It Could Be Worse

*When you put the OJ in the laundry room...just laugh.

*When you find the match to that earring you just threw out under wet receipts and an orange peel in the car's drink holder...just laugh.

*When you run out of gas in the middle of a left turn and tell the officer that your other half is on the way with gas AND blurt out, "I've already got a ticket for the expired plates," before he even notices...just laugh.

*When you find yourself knee deep in laundry, with a counter full of dishes, jewelry supplies engulfing the dining room, reptile supplies in the bathtub and a kitchen table covered in stacks of bills, take-out menus, advertisements for things you

want to do and a miscellaneous shoe box full of crap that doesn't really belong anywhere just as company arrives...just laugh.

*When you hear, "You're funny without your pill, Mummy"...just laugh.

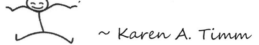

~ Karen A. Timm

Karen A. Timm, Elementary School Vice-Principal has ADHD, is dedicated to educating herself and others about succeeding with neurodiversity; loves her fabulous child with ADHD.
@ADHDinPrincipal

Neurodiversity: It's How You Frame It!

Hyperactive ⇒ Full of Energy

Strong Willed ⇒ Tenacious/ Persistent

Day Dreamer ⇒ Creative/ Imaginative

Dare Devil ⇒ Risk Taker/ Adventurous

Aggressive ⇒ Assertive

Question Authority ⇒ Independent Thinker

Lazy ⇒ Laid Back/ Relaxed

Talkative ⇒ Enthusiastic

Argumentative ⇒ Persuasive

Forgetful ⇒ Hyperfocused/ Deeply absorbed

Manipulative ⇒ Delegates Well

Bossy ⇒ Signs of Leadership

Distractible ⇒ Curious

~ *Cindy Goldrich, EdM, ACAC*

Cindy Goldrich, EdM, ACAC, ADHD Parent Coach, Teacher Trainer, and author of 8 Keys to Parenting Children with ADHD
www.PTScoaching.com Cindy@PTScoaching.com (516) 802-0593

Coffee Pot Alarm Clocks

Like many people in college, waking up and getting out of bed for morning classes can be a near impossibility. Setting traditional alarms often fail. One innovative ADHD college student came up with his own way of making sure he didn't miss any of his morning classes. Each night, he would prepare the coffee and set the automatic timer to go off in the morning. Then he would set his alarm by his bed to go off five minutes before the coffee pot. His fail-proof system? When he made the coffee, he made sure that the coffee carafe was not under the coffee maker. If he didn't get up shortly after his bedside alarm went off, the coffee would end up all over the floor! According to him, it never failed. Wacky often works!

~Laurie Dupar, PMHNP, RN, PCC

Laurie Dupar, PMHNP, RN, PCC is a trained Psychiatric Nurse Practitioner and 12 year veteran ADHD coach specializing in mentoring and training emerging ADHD Coaches. www.coachingforadhd.com support@coachingforadhd.com

ADHD and Lost Jewelry

I have a drawer full of single earrings. I can't seem to let go of them; gold, silver, jewels, all are so dear, so precious and SO alone.

I have found many techniques for not losing jewelry; the secret of course is to create a system and actually use it! This is where mindfulness comes in.

But first, a eulogy in memoriam to that which I loved and lost: A VERY expensive 3 jeweled drop earring (an amazing sale no less) wrapped in tissue in my jean pocket because my ear hurt. I forgot about it, checked my pockets before doing laundry (I give myself credit here folks), but threw away the tissue.

A mother-of-pearl/gold elephant necklace sent to me by a dear friend. The clasp was loose, but I hurriedly listened to the "Yeah Buts" instead of my "Gut Instinct." It fell off at my office (after checking it repeatedly) and no one turned it in. It was an impulsive vs. mindful decision. I didn't stop to breathe (and think it through) before WANTING to wear it. So many more precious pieces with memories for each, but I'll stop there (p.s., don't buy cheap gold chains!).

My mother was fond of saying that I always 'learned my lesson the hard way.' Now when I clean or put my earrings in I always pull up the stopper first in the bathroom sink. When my ear hurts in the middle of the night I no longer put the earring under my pillow (never to be seen again), but in a tiny bowl on the nightstand. If I take them out when I'm not at home they go in a zip compartment in my wallet (NOT in the change part!). Rings go in a tiny bowl on the microwave.

I will confess that I now tend to obsessively check the clip on the posts to make sure they're resting tightly against my ears. Why, you may ask, do you even wear earrings? Well, I actually stopped for a few years when my frustration level was maxed out. But, the more I meditated, breathed purposefully throughout the day and practiced mindfulness, the more I knew that I was ready to decorate my ears once again. I'm even confident enough to wear my mom's ruby earrings.

If I can keep track of my jewelry, I KNOW that you can too!

Always remember, mindfulness matters.

~ Judi Jerome, LICSW, LADC

Judi Jerome, LICSW, LADC, owner of Mindfulness Matters Coaching in Vermont, is a Coach, Psychotherapist, Consultant, Writer and Speaker specializing in coaching adults, professionals, business owners, physicians, and graduate students with AD/HD or similar life challenges. Judi teaches mindfulness meditation and believes that with mindfulness everyone has potential within to achieve success beyond the current limits that problems such as distractibility, time management, disorganization, morning madness and late night hyper-focusing may be imposing on their lives. Her motto – Empowerment, growth and maintenance for positive life changes. Read all about Judi's coaching, her blog, published articles and book reviews at www.judijerome.com

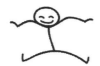

"I prefer to distinguish ADD as attention abundance disorder. Everything is just so interesting...remarkably at the same time."

~ Frank Coppola, MA, ODC, ACG

You Yelled – Get to the Jar!

It's not easy keeping things calm all the time. Every now and then, someone yells and things get out of hand. When that happens, usually all hope of reasoning and problem solving dissolve. So next time you or your kid yells instead of talking, try this:

Have a large jar (preferably not glass!) and have each family member fill it with about 5 tasks or actions. Next time someone yells, they must take a slip of paper from the jar and perform the required task.

Examples:

   15 push-ups

   Bang drum sticks on a pillow

   Run around the block

Use thick crayons to draw a picture

Exercise and action can reduce the tension. The idea here is to calm things down so that the real issue causing the stress and anger can be dealt with.

~ Cindy Goldrich, EdM, ACAC

Cindy Goldrich, EdM, ACAC, is an ADHD Parent Coach, Teacher Trainer, and author of 8 Keys to Parenting Children with ADHD www.PTScoaching.com Cindy@PTScoaching.com (516) 802-0593

My Career with ADHD - A Simple Love Story

In my teens and twenties I worked as a retail clerk and secretary.

A lawyer I worked for wanted me to write personal letters and mail her Christmas presents. I staunchly refused to do so. I did not enjoy taking orders or feeling subservient to anyone. I often made silly mistakes like copying the wrong documents.

I was fired over and over, so I worked as a "temp" to lessen the pressure. Yet the loss of jobs in my twenties resulted in low self-confidence. Why was this happening? In 2008, I was diagnosed with ADHD. It took almost thirty years to finally know why.

Failing to understand the kind of work that suited me after college graduation, I returned to secretarial work for the next four years. I call these my lost years and felt depressed.

I was convinced that to do what I wanted, I had to become "professional" in something. Being a "professional" meant freedom from judgments, criticism, menial tasks and feeling crappy about myself. I had to somehow show the world my greatest assets, not knowing exactly what they were.

My rebellious nature was untamed in those days. I did not like answering to anyone. I was destined to find a way to work independently. I still balk at taking orders, although less so. The anxiety of being "found out" was overwhelming back then. I felt like a fraud.

Out of sheer determination and fear, I pushed myself to get a Masters in Vocational Counseling. My graduate degree would be flexible and marketable for years to come. I liked that the work had a beginning, middle and end, with a spiritual element. Most importantly, it still represents who I am. It allows me to keep things interesting, fun and exciting.

As far back as I can remember, I have had a strong desire to help people. In my first career, I was a vocational rehabilitation counselor. But after 10 years, I began to burn out. For those of us with ADHD, job burnout is often the kiss of career death.

I became resentful of the players in the system I worked within, and the roles they played. I no longer enjoyed the reporting aspect of this work. I no longer liked taking insurance people to lunch or keeping track of my time. The clients were often angry. I liked motivated clients.

I was unhappy. I wanted something that I looked forward to doing. I got additional training in career counseling and

coaching, and twenty-five years later still love it.

So why am I sharing this story? Because I was one of the lucky ones who was stubborn enough to make sure I got the education and training to do what I loved. My ADHD was clearly the reason for my fierce determination.

I help people and change lives. I am never bored. I choose the environment I want to work in. I make my own hours. I meet great people in a wide variety of careers. I appreciate careers I would never dream of doing. I teach, train, counsel, coach, write, public speak, create, synthesize and coordinate interesting information. I use all the skills I love in the fields I am most fascinated with - education and counseling.

There is much more to this story. The bottom line is the work I am doing now fits my life with ADHD. No matter how far I stray, I keep coming back.

I hope this knowledge helps you make a long term, exciting career decision that evolves over time. This is my prayer for you.

~ Shell Mendelson, MS, Career Coach for Adults with ADHD

With over 25 years of experience and education in the career counseling and coaching arena, Shell Mendelson has helped hundreds of clients make successful career transitions. Shell brings counseling, coaching, teaching, training and nurturing gifts to help clients FOCUS on defining, illuminating, creating and transforming lack of clarity to a well-defined career or business choice for adults with ADHD. Diagnosed in 2008, Shell has a deep awareness of how ADHD impacts your work experience. A 40-year proven System designed for ADHD Adults keeps it simple. Shell is the founder and former CEO of KidzArt, an international franchise system. http://www.shellmendelson.com   shell.mendelson@gmail.com

Did You Wake up on the "Bad Side" of Your Brain?

You know that saying, "I woke up on the wrong side of the bed?" With ADHD, we have days when it feels like we have woken up on "the bad side of the brain." Just getting out of bed is an accomplishment, and feels overwhelming.

On bad brain days, try these:

- Get up, even if you don't feel like it.
- Continue your daily routines: eat, shower, dress, and take your medication.
- Call in the troops: hang with supportive friends and family.

- Be kind to yourself. Treat yourself to a latte, favorite place, or movie.
- Ask yourself what might have contributed to your "bad side of the brain" day. Did you sleep poorly, change diet or skip your medication? Are you stressed? Address the issue.

Use these strategies to minimize the impact of a "bad side of the brain" day, and remember: there's always tomorrow!

~Laurie Dupar, PMHNP, RN, PCC

Laurie Dupar, PMHNP, RN, PCC is a trained Psychiatric Nurse Practitioner and 12 year veteran ADHD coach specializing in mentoring and training emerging ADHD Coaches.
www.coachingforadhd.com   support@coachingforadhd.com

??ADHD or ADHD or ADHDDH!!

TTENTION DEFICIT HYPERACTIVITY DISORDER

Gibberish Nonsense – Green Growing Red

Yellow Laces Calling – From My Bed

Beholding Dreams – Diamonds Or Lead

Kaleidoscope Sites – Nothing To Dread

Gibberish Solutions – Sensing In My Head

Extraordinary Is Extraordinary

Tis Me – Tis You

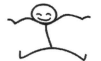

Gibberish Is Gibberish

Sense Is Sense

ADHD Is ADHD

? What Are We !

Tis Our Riddle

Here Is How I Solve My Riddle

Attention Deficit Hyperactivity Disorder

A Captive Life – I - ???

My Soul Wandering My Soul

Amidst My Fractured Bits And My Disconnects

In My Somewhere Of My Nowhere

Relentless Restless Restrained Reaching

srewsnA roF snoitseuQ gniyoJ sgnidnE dnoyeB

Exploring Explosive Expressive Exquisite

Chaos Celebrating Chasing Creations

Crazy Sense Senseless Sane

Dream Thought Being

My Soul Finding My Soul

!!! - I – A Life Master

Attention Different Highly Driven

Emae

I celebrate gibberish as opportunities to make sense out of nonsense

I see myself and everyone else as extraordinary

I live not as disordered but as driven

Do you make sense of your gibberish?

Do you live your extraordinary gifts?

Is your ADHD – disordered or Driven

ATTENTION DIFFERENT HIGHLY DRIVEN

One of the extraordinary gifts is our ability to dream beyond horizons

Attention Different Highly Driven Dreaming Beyond Horizons

ADHD / ADHDDH

Dream with me a bit

Sense the sense of what I dream

Dream of a world beyond our horizons

Rule number ten in my rules of life is that there are no rules

For to pursue a life of Health is to pursue a life of Peace

Health is the thread that weaves the Tapestries of Our lives

Self – Others – World

There is nothing more essential to what happens in Our lives than Our Health

There is nothing more important to what happens to Our Health

There is nothing more powerful to what happens to Our Health

Than what We individually do about Our own Health

Than what We collectively do about Everyone's Health

Dream of Health this way

Health is Your true Wealth

The extent of Your Wealth of Tapestries

Is measured by the strength of the Thread of Your Health

Live life richly with a Wealth of Your Health

Accumulate a treasure chest of the ten precious metals and stones of

WORLD CLASS HEALTH

Maintain A Healthy Weight

Avoid Self Abusive Behaviors

Take Time And Restore

Prevent Your Preventable Medical Problems

Control Your Controllable Medical Problems

GOLD: Eat Healthy

SILVER: Exercise

BRONZE, RUBY, EMERALD,

SAPPHIRE, OPAL, PLATINUM

Use Your Family's Medical History To Fine Tune Your Health Efforts

Who Knows How To Guide Your Health

Share Health Forward

PEARL: Have A Health Guide

DIAMOND

(A Dreamer's Paradise - A world of Health where everyone everyday tries

To better their own Health and the Health of those around them

Based on Catherine Ryan Hyde's "Pay It Forward")

ADHD or not, imagine the wealth of tapestries

In simply living the simple principles of

World Class Health

Imagine the wonder of a world all life could joy

If we tried to better our Health And the Health of those around us

EveryOne EveryDay

Start Everyday With Please

Mirror Mirror On The Wall

Who Will Make Me Healthiest Of All

Roses Are Red My Friend, Violets Are Blue

Your Health My Friend, Is All About You Fixing You

Roses Are Red, Sunflowers Are Yellow

Go Out And Help Fix Some Other Fellow

Then Take The Pledge Of Health

And Remember As Well While Fixing Yourself

My Health is My responsibility and I swear to make some effort everyday

To better My Health and the Health of those around Me

ATTENTION DIFFERENT HIGHLY DRIVEN DREAMING BEYOND HORIZONS

Thanks For Dreaming With Me

~ Michael Alan Schuler MD

Michael Alan Schuler MD A Colorful Spinning Top - Attention Different Highly Driven - (ADHD) A former Cleveland Clinic Wooster, Ohio - Internist, Pulmonologist, Intensivist He remains in Wooster - Celebrating his retirement years With Pat - The Life who allows him the privilege of being her husband He thinks of himself as an Artist and Writer ECHOES AND SHADOWS CHASING LIGHT Is a colorful spin of some of his unique views on Life, Family, Health, America, God, ADHD and who knows what else He is still trying to figure it out (2012 The Wooster Book Company, Ohio - www.woosterbook.com) You can message Mike at echoesandshadows1212@yahoo.com

Sanity Restored

When a day unfolds with a boatload of ADHD challenges, I reach for Mindfulness and heaping doses of Self-Compassion. Recently, I arrived home without my keys! No worries, the landlord will let me in.

Later, I began some online banking, but couldn't find my bank card. I thought, "it's in my coat, but where's my coat?" I'm thinking, great, now all 3 are missing! Momentary pause, deep breath in and out. I'll deal with this tomorrow. Before bed, I opened a letter stating I owed the bank and landlord $70!

Again, deep breath in and out! The following day I retrieved all 3 items and the bank and landlord reimbursed my $70! Accepting things as they are in the present moment with a healthy dose of Self-Compassion can be just the antidote to restoring my sanity for yet another day.

~ Veronica Taylor, Life Coach (CTI)

Veronica Taylor, Life Coach, Mindfulness Proponent, Meditation Facilitator, Neuroscience Enthusiast, working with Clients to unleash their gifts and talents to help them Shine!
veronica.taylor@sympatico.ca

Don't Forget the Fun!

Let's be honest: Parenting an ADHD child is a wonderful, exhilarating challenge. We can be so overwhelmed with the chaos, the reminders (of reminders of reminders), the problems at school, etc. that we forget to take a moment and have fun. Often ADHD kids love to celebrate and have fun, and it can be for anything. A touchdown scored on the football field, a grade on a test, or the fact that it's a Wednesday can be cause for celebration. So what do we do to make sure we can still get things done that need to get done? We can create time in our schedules to celebrate. That doesn't mean a big blow out party every week, but it means recognizing and celebrating those things that are meaningful to our kiddos.

~ Jared and DeAnn Jennette

Jared and DeAnn Jennette are trained coaches who specialize in families of adopted children with ADHD, SPD and other "alphabet soup" diagnoses. embraceparentcoaching@gmail.com www.embraceparentcoaching.com

Time to Play (Everyday)!

Research shows that young children lose attention in class if recess is delayed and conversely, both attitudes toward learning and test scores improve when significant school time is spent on art, music and physical activity.

Research also shows that "green time" – time out in nature – benefits kids with ADHD, as well as all of us. And experiences of awe and laughter benefit our physical and mental health, even expanding our sense of time.

So, consider these questions:

• What is play for you? How regularly do you incorporate play into your week?

• How often do you get outside in nature? When could you increase this?

• What makes you laugh? What might help you laugh more?

• What gives you a feeling of awe? Might any spiritual/religious practices, artwork or natural beauty help you tap into this more often?

Most importantly: what are you waiting for?

~ *Elizabeth (Liz) Ahmann, ScD, RN, ACC*

ADHD Coach, Liz Ahmann, ScD, RN, ACC, coaches using evidence-based approaches and teaches mindfulness classes for individuals with ADHD. Learn more at www.lizahmann.com www.lizahmann.com/mindfulness.html

Whine Your Way to a Happy Career with ADHD

Here's how: Draw a line down the middle of a piece of paper - left side (-), right side (+).

In the (-) category on the left, make a list of EVERYTHING in your past jobs you did not like or you were resistant to doing. Complaining is OK!

On the (-) list put every task, skill, characteristics of people who made you crazy, environment (cubical? ugly building?), product you sold or made that you were embarrassed to tell anyone about, etc.

Now take the (-) side and decide what the opposite of each item is for you – in other words put what you would prefer on the (+) side of each item (i.e. people who micromanage (-) to people who are supportive (+)). Prioritize them in order of preference. What stands out?

Congrats! You have just clarified a few of the most critical elements in your life's work!

~ Shell Mendelson, MS, Career Coach for Adults with ADHD

Shell Mendelson, MS, Career Coach for Adults with ADHD helps clients go from chaos to focused career choice with unparalleled planning and support. www.shellmendelson.com shell.mendelson@gmail.com

"If a man does not keep pace with his companions, perhaps it is because he

hears a different drummer. Let him step to the music, which he hears, however measured or far away."

~ Henry David Thoreau

 ## Sing and Dance Your Way Through Any Task

I'm a musician with ADHD. Often I turn to music in times of stress, anxiety, or even boring jobs. Music is a great help when ADHD gets in my way.

I'm a child of the '60s and '70s, so when I have a big task to do or am feeling stressed, I put on a "Greatest Hits" CD – maybe The Beatles, Linda Ronstadt, Elton John or Chicago.

Most CDs run around 70 minutes. Once one is playing, I can clean the linen closet, sort through old clothes, find outdated magazines to trash or donate, clean out a kitchen cupboard or go digital and download a special playlist for a specific task. This is my time to SING (at the top of my lungs) and DANCE (boogie, funky, whatever). Before I know it, the task is complete and I feel great!

~ *Valerie C Krupp*

Valerie Krupp, BMEd, MALS, is an ADHD Coach who helps adult clients put the puzzle pieces of ADHD together to create their best life. Visit her at ADDultLifeCoaching.com (803) 413-7398

First: Attention - Then: Directions

My husband and I learned early on that some things got our sons' attention, and some things did not. If we wanted them to follow directions, it worked best to sing rather than speak the direction. We'd make up songs like "Baby, get your coat on. It's time to go." My husband was a very good singer. I am not. We had a joke that I would stop singing when they did what was requested. They told me they would close their eyes, and settle for bed, if only I would stop with the lullaby! Now, as adults, when they get stuck in an emotion like frustration, if I sing, they stop and laugh, breaking the hold of the emotion.

~ Pat Corbett, BEd, MC, MSW

Pat Corbett (Calgary) is an in-home family support worker at Connections Counseling and Consulting and facilitator at Columbia College. Her dream: bridging gaps. www.reframingthebox.com

Bright Shiny Coach Syndrome©

ADHD coaching is fast being recognized as a key in experiencing long-lasting success with ADHD. Sometimes it is easy to get distracted by prices or get swept up in another's credentials. Choosing the right coach for you or your child is important. Here are some questions to consider:

- What are their certifications/credentials in coaching?
- Where/how did they get their ADHD expertise?

- What is this coach's specialty (parenting, college, child)? Does it match your needs?

- How will this coach monitor my progress?

- What are the sessions like?

- Do they work in person, over the phone, or using Skype? Does this work for me?

Finally, the "gut response" question: "Do I want to work with this coach?" Coaching is a partnership, and feeling like you connect with your coach and they "get" you, may be the tie breaker.

~Laurie Dupar, PMHNP, RN, PCC

Laurie Dupar, PMHNP, RN, PCC is a trained Psychiatric Nurse Practitioner and 12 year veteran ADHD coach specializing in mentoring and training emerging ADHD Coaches. www.coachingforadhd.com support@coachingforadhd.com

A Spoonful of Sugar

My son realized I was different whenever he got sick. While other moms might peek in once in a while, I'd check in every 10-15 minutes. I checked for discomfort, temperature, skin, eyes, ounces of fluid drank and brought a remedy... for boredom (the greatest fear for someone with ADHD).

Instead of reading him a story, I came in with 10 comic books (each a different superhero) and diverse projects requiring several skills and tools—metal tapping artwork, cutting and painting frames for pictures and assembling intricate models. Once he was well, he busted out of Mom's Rehab with an entire new collection of gifts for friends and family. My little elf!

Sometimes I worried he had no time for rest, but he assured me he felt he was a lucky kid. His mom showed him that any experience, even being sick, could have an element of fun.

~ Angelis Iglesias, HSP, HSS, ADHD Coach, Consultant, Researcher

Angelis Iglesias, HSP, HSS, ADHD Coach, Researcher. Technology, Social Media for Coaches Faculty Impact Coaching Academy.
www.mindheartinstitute.com www.angelisiglesias.com
ai@angelisiglesias.com

What, Me Study?

Going back to school later in life after being diagnosed with ADHD is a challenging adventure. The key for me is getting academic accommodations, and developing my own quirky study methods.

My Inattentive-type ADHD makes processing and reading comprehension difficult. It helps to have fewer notes on each page. I take notes by hand, turn my notebook sideways, and write in large capital letters that fill the page with fewer words.

I use colored pens to highlight key words. Next I record my notes on my phone, speaking slowly, repeating key phrases, and leaving long pauses. Finally, I commit the information to memory by listening while doing household tasks! When listening back I have time to recall and speak the answers aloud. This extra effort pays off tremendously!

Don't try this alone!

I connected with two other students in my dreaded anatomy and physiology courses, dreaded because it required a lot of (boring!) memorization, a challenge for ADHDers. Our study group met weekly for 2-4 hours to work on assignments and take turns quizzing each other and trying to explain the complicated material. Eventually we gained a deeper understanding of the material and new perspectives on how to approach it.

Our group also served as a place where we could cheer each other on whenever we felt frustrated or overwhelmed. Studying regularly with others increased my productivity, accountability, and confidence. Later, the three of us met regularly to study for the GRE and work on the applications to our respective graduate programs.

Can't think? Discover Your Inner Artist and Soar!

I used to have a narrow idea of what success looked like. Discovering painting has helped in ways I never imagined. I thought that the painting class prerequisite for my desired master's degree would be embarrassing at best. Instead I found that the bright colors and the varied movement of the brushstrokes improved my executive functioning! Today, after painting for even just a few minutes, my brain is more focused, alert and ready to work on difficult things. Painting was new and exciting yet meditative. It has become my primary way for dealing with academic anxiety. Discovering my inner artist and giving myself permission to do things my wacky way has made life and school easier. As Ralph Waldo Emerson said, "To be yourself in a world that is constantly trying to make you something else is the greatest accomplishment."

~ Ariel Davis, ADHD Coach

Ariel Davis is an ADHD coach and Occupational Therapy Master's Candidate, specializing in teens and adults. Her strengths-based, sensory-focused approach is based in her experience supporting people with addiction, ADHD and other mental health issues, as well as her work in the creative arts. Connect with her: www.ADHDstrengthscoach.com ADHDstrengthscoach@gmail.com

Are You a Helicopter <u>Partner</u>?

D o you hover over your spouse while they're doing tasks? Does your nagging, pleading and anger fail to motivate? If so, you may be a helicopter partner!

While helicopter partners are borne from frustration when job after job isn't completed, the problem is helicoptering doesn't build respect...or allow your partner to learn what works and what doesn't.

So, try these tips:

1. Remind your partner only once. Nagging isn't sexy!

2. Leave it. Just because you can do it, doesn't mean you should.

3. Don't take responsibility for your partner's actions.

4. Let your partner fail. That's the best way to learn!

5. Don't do for your partner what they can do for themselves. .

Remember you're building a healthy, equal partner-ship you both can enjoy for years to come.

~Laurie Dupar, PMHNP, RN, PCC

Laurie Dupar, PMHNP, RN, PCC is a trained Psychiatric Nurse Practitioner and 12 year veteran ADHD coach specializing in mentoring and training emerging ADHD Coaches. www.coachingforadhd.com support@coachingforadhd.com

Lock Away Success

Years ago, S.C. Johnson and son had a contest to see who had the best idea for using their Ziploc© bags. Now, with so many different sizes and shapes, there is no end to the ingenious ways to use these handy plastic bags with the sealable tops when you have ADHD. Here are some of my favorites:

- Makeup bag

- School supply bag for pencils, pens, sticky notes

- Tablet protector while cooking

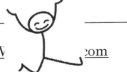

- Shoe storage and protector

- Junk drawer organizers

- Bag to keep medications in

- Phone protector if you might be in the rain, near water, sand or a little one with sticky fingers

- Cord organizer

- Clothes organizer for each day of travel. (Doubles as dirty clothes bag at the end of the day!)

What are some ways you use these bags? Please let me know at: Stephanie@bridgingyourworldstogether.com

~ Stephanie J. Noel Kirlin, ADHD Coach

Stephanie J. Noel Kirlin, Executive, Leadership, Group and ADHD Coach in Santa Barbara, CA. Helps clients find clarity, joy and achieve personal success. www.bridgingyourworldstogether.com Stephanie@bridgingyourworldstogether.com

What's Emoji Got to Do with It?

When I'm coaching my ADHD clients, we have fun! They come in stressed that they're not measuring up. I turn that right around! I share that I'm ADHD, too. ADHD is the magic that makes us uniquely creative. We just need to harness and direct that energy in creative ways.

One client is starting a dog training business. We use bright red, dog paw emojis in our daily texts, to make her tasks more appealing. She sets three goals a day and sends me Emoji check marks and dog paws when she accomplishes them. Everyone loves rewards! I give her Starbuck's cards for weekly check-ins.

Success can be exciting and empowering if you have a buddy! ADHD coaches are buddies. I'm thrilled to see how happy my clients are when they reach their goals, one fun step at a time!

~ Candace Sahm, MA Ed

Candace Sahm, MA Ed, ADHD Coach and Special Educator with JST Coach training. Supports youth and adults to reach their highest potential. www.candacesahm.com   coachcandace1@gmail.com 301-229-9515

"I like nonsense, it wakes up the brain cells."

~ Dr. Seuss

Be Imperfect on Purpose

If logic, conventional wisdom, or your relatives' advice isn't working, just stop following it and stop beating yourself up for being imperfect.

In fact, start being imperfect on purpose!

In my practice, I find that many parents are doing too much, not too little! They're doing everything they can think of and then are so frustrated and demoralized when it doesn't work.

It's time to give yourself a break. Declare an "Imperfect Day," when your whole family has to do everything imperfectly, or 28 or 6 things imperfectly. Or you all get to be imperfect from 2pm to 8pm.

Wear a tutu and cowboy boots, eat soup with a fork, go get ice cream in your PJs, do your kids' chores for them, but imperfectly! Highlight your imperfection in photos and videos!

Balance the challenges with joy and laughter to nurture your ADHD family's heart.

~ *Margit Crane Luria, MA, MS, MEd*

A 30-year teacher and school counselor, Margit Crane Luria's current work guides ADHD families through behavior and/or executive function challenges. www.GiftedWithADD.com

Hidden Highlights

As an ADHD coach, some of my favorite clients are college students. Students are hard working and persistent. Reading, lots of reading, is a big part of college. The volume of reading can be overwhelming, not to mention uninteresting. And uninteresting material is a big potential pitfall for many students. One clever student created the following strategy to keep herself focused and interested when doing assigned reading. When she first read through a text, she would highlight everything in yellow. Doing this helped her keep track of what she had read. Next, she would go back and highlight key pieces in blue, which turned green when put over the yellow, or with pink, which would also change colors. This use of creative combinations of colors was fun, engaging and helped her keep on track with an otherwise painstaking job.

~Laurie Dupar, PMHNP, RN, PCC

Laurie Dupar, PMHNP, RN, PCC is a trained Psychiatric Nurse Practitioner and 12 year veteran ADHD coach specializing in mentoring and training emerging ADHD Coaches. www.coachingforadhd.com support@coachingforadhd.com

ADD Yin Yang

My husband, Dennis thinks clearly and acts decisively. A buttoned-up corporate guy, Dennis is a crew cut. I'm kinky, blond hair. He's calm to my internal and external chaos.

Politically correct (to a fault), Dennis delivers bad news so politely, you miss it. Not the case with me. "I really don't like spending time with you," I recently said to a relative. What?!

Dennis is goal-oriented and disciplined. He finds a 6-mile running course wherever we travel while I'm looking for the dessert course.

I don't have a brain that allows me to act like Dennis. So I did the next best thing and acquired one through marriage. I'm the Yin to his Yang. Our opposite brains have created strife in our 25-year marriage, but I think we're in our Zen Zone.

Dennis is my rock, and he says I'm his star. Together, we're a Yin Yang Rock Star couple.

~ Zion Banks, ZB Media Consulting

Zion Banks is a media consultant and thriving ADDer. Zion's pride points: wife (25 years) and mom (3 girls). She calls her ADHD diagnosis "freeing."

Just Breathe: Self-Regulation for Parents

Let's deal with the elephant in the room (or on the page in this case): Our ADHD kids can have some serious meltdowns. Those meltdowns can be for things big or small, but when they happen, it usually takes over the whole house. Often, the sterner we get, the worse the meltdown can get.

How do we keep things from getting worse? We have to keep our cool, or as we call it, "self-regulate." Our children can't do what we can't do ourselves, so if we want them to regulate, we have to keep ourselves regulated. How? One way is to take a deep breath. Deep breathing has been proven to release oxytocin, a hormone that calms us down and decreases the level of cortisol in our brain. So when you recognize the meltdown, make sure you calm yourself first so you can help your child calm down.

~ Jared and DeAnn Jennette, Parent Coaches

Jared and DeAnn Jennette are trained coaches who specialize in families of adopted children with ADHD, SPD, and other "alphabet soup" diagnoses. www.embraceparentcoaching.com embraceparentcoaching@gmail.com

Mindfulness for ADHD? No Way!

"It's impossible for me to sit still that long."

"You expect me to clear my mind? Are you kidding?"

"There's no way I could stick with a habit like meditating."

People with ADHD are embracing the idea that mindfulness could help them to feel less ADHD. Trouble is they also embrace the idea that mindfulness would be impossible for them.

What is needed is an ADHD-Informed approach:

• Start with short practices.

• Use both being still and moving meditations.

• End with honoring your practice.

• Use reminders, cues, and other external supports.

• Enlist a mindfulness buddy.

• Don't try to force your mind to be blank – simply notice thoughts and watch them pass.

• Don't worry if you think you're no good at meditating. The important word in mindfulness practice is practice.

When you feel like mindfulness might be impossible for you, try an ADHD-informed approach.

~ *Casey Dixon, SCAC, BCC, MSEd*

Casey Dixon is Success Strategist and ADHD Coach for www.mindfullyadd.com and www.dixonlifecoaching.com, employing a unique focus on science-based, innovative strategies for demand-ridden professionals with ADHD.

Do You Brush Your Teeth?

Yes . . . that's right . . . do you brush your teeth? This question may seem random in a strategy book for ADHD, but whether or not you brush your teeth is a good indicator of your ability to learn other new habits.

Brushing our teeth is not a natural act. It neither keeps us safe from predators nor adds nutritional sustenance. Hand-eye coordination is required to do it properly. It takes time, and it requires organizing--water, toothpaste and toothbrush. Yet, most of us learn to complete brushing our teeth every day.

Tooth brushing is a great example of how, with practice, we can learn a new behavior or habit.

So, the next time you feel discouraged, and wonder if you can learn a new habit, ask yourself, "Did I brush my teeth today?" And, there's your answer!

~Laurie Dupar, PMHNP, RN, PCC

Laurie Dupar, PMHNP, RN, PCC is a trained Psychiatric Nurse Practitioner and 12 year veteran ADHD coach specializing in mentoring and training emerging ADHD Coaches.
www.coachingforadhd.com support@coachingforadhd.com

Tag-I'm It!

I have always been able to amuse and entertain myself, and still do as a twenty-something college student. Rather than just fidgeting and twitching, I will do some sort of physical activity when I'm able. With friends, it often turns into a game ending in laughter and amusement for the whole group. I find we take ourselves too seriously so often that every now and then it's fun to just do something "childish." Even in college, games of Red Rover and Duck-Duck-Goose are favorite ways to use my fidgety energy. I use it as a way to have fun with those around me. I have to learn you're never too old for a "childlike" game and everyone else seems to secretly love them too! Someone with a playful impulse or creative idea just has to get things started.

~ Dr. Billi Bittan

Dr. Billi, PhD, certified Co-active ADHD Coach and Neuro-Cognitive Behavioral Therapist, is the founder of AttentionB and creator of the LEVERAGE ADHD™ System. www.attentionb.com

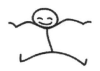 # The Day Frogs Flew

The Ferguson family was heading off 'down south' for their annual holiday. Everybody was looking forward to arriving at the destination. Nobody was looking forward to the four-hour drive it would take to get there. The route was scenic, the car was comfortable, but three children with ADHD confined to the back seat meant sibling conflict on steroids.

Father Ferguson had stooped shoulders as he sat down behind the wheel, remembering the constant bickering in the back seat last time they had driven to their holiday. Mother Ferguson, however, was smiling, as she calmly unveiled her secret weapon - a bag of individually wrapped Freddo Frogs – every Australian kid's favorite chocolate treat. She explained to their three children that they would be allowed to eat every Freddo Frog in the bag when they arrived at their destination, on condition that they refrained from bickering during the trip. Mr. 9 year-old swiftly calculated that 12 Freddo Frogs translated to 4 treats each, which was more chocolate than they had eaten since Easter. Harmony prevailed as the car pulled out.

Thirty minutes into the journey, Ms. 7yo accused Mr. 9yo of leaning too closely into her space, and the fragile peace shattered as all hell broke loose on the back seat. Mother

Ferguson calmly took one Freddo Frog out of the bag, removed its wrapper, and held it up for the children to see it in all of its chocolaty splendor. You could have heard a pin drop as she opened her window and tossed the frog to the wind. This caused a near riot, with Ms. 11yo telling her younger siblings off for ruining their treat, Mr. 9yo informing Ms. 7yo that she would only get 3 Freddos because it was all her fault, and Ms. 7yo retorting that it wouldn't have happened in the first place if he hadn't been BREATHING HER AIR! Father Ferguson's shoulders stooped lower.

Mother Ferguson, still smiling, did not say a word. She merely repeated the process, as another chocolate frog became road kill, and then another.

And then it became quiet. Ms. 11yo popped her headphones on and started listening to her new audio book. Mr. 9yo asked Ms. 7yo to help him count yellow cars. Father Ferguson sat up straight and grinned. The holiday had begun!

~ Dr. Michele Toner, PhD, PCC, PCAC

Dr. Michele Toner, PhD, PCC, PCAC, is based in Western Australia, and coaches people from around the world. Her Masters and PhD research, coupled with 20 years of hands-on experience make her well equipped to empower her clients, as they learn to conquer the chaos and stay in control. She works with individuals and their families to identify and harness their strengths, address their challenges, and make ADHD 'work for them.' As a registered mentor coach, Michele also empowers new coaches to be the best they can. www.micheletoner.com

"I'm sorry...I wasn't paying attention to what I was thinking."

~ Shelley Curtiss

Finding Fun

When the boys were preschoolers, I chose to shop at department stores or grocery stores that had a toy section. We would find the items we needed to buy and then take the cart to the toy section. We lived on a tight budget and did not often buy toys. We would take some time to talk about the toys on the shelf - the color of the shield or outfit a particular action figure had. We'd talk about what the toys might be dreaming of as they sat on the shelf. Toys had to stay on the shelf, but our imaginations could take them anywhere. To this day, my boys still "window shop" and plan what they want to save their money for.

~ Pat Corbett, BEd, MC, MSW

Pat Corbett (Calgary) is an in-home family support worker at Connections Counseling and Consulting and facilitator at Columbia College. Her dream: bridging gaps. www.reframingthebox.com

Do You Suffer from Time Zone Dyscalculia?

In today's world, scheduling calls, meetings or appointments in different time zones is common. Keeping track of them accurately can be a nightmare! In fact, I am sure I have what I fondly call "time zone dyscalculia!" I always ended up miscalculating the hours and inevitably called at the wrong time. In order to keep my client's sanity and mine, I came up with the strategies below:

- Check out smart phone apps for "time zone calculators."
- Keep a "time zone map" handy.
- Use an online appointment-scheduling system (www.scheduleonce.com is my favorite).
- Set some old-fashioned wall clocks to the most common time zones you work with.

Never suffer from Time Zone Dyscalculia again!

~Laurie Dupar, ADHD Mentor and Trainer

Laurie Dupar, PMHNP, RN, PCC is a trained Psychiatric Nurse Practitioner and 12 year veteran ADHD coach specializing in mentoring and training emerging ADHD Coaches.
www.coachingforadhd.com support@coachingforadhd.com

Tipping into Technology

No doubt technology is an ADHDer's best friend. Sometimes I think all the gadgets, apps and gizmos were created with us especially in mind. Along with the obvious uses, here are some tech tips you might not have considered:

• Always buy the computer/smartphone/iPod with the most memory.

• Pace while listening to audio books if you are a kinesthetic learner.

• iPhone® now has the option to add the travel time to your calendar appointment.

• Set your phone timer before you step into the shower to remind you when to get out.

• Chronos© is an app that shows you how and where you spend your time. You set goals and the app automatically tracks your progress, then emails you weekly with the results.

• Unstuck© is an app that utilizes cognitive behavioral therapy principles and cards with questions to get your ADHD brain unstuck.

~ Stephanie J. Noel Kirlin, ADHD Coach

Stephanie J. Noel Kirlin, Executive, Leadership, Group & ADHD Coach in Santa Barbara, CA. Helps clients find clarity, passion and achieve personal success. www.bridgingyourworldstogether.com Stephanie@bridgingyourworldstogether.com

What Do You Mean, Focus?

Research shows it's actually possible to train yourself to focus better. Surprisingly, one way to do this is by purposely noticing your distractions...and then returning to whatever you had intended to do.

Here's an example of how this mindful re-focusing works:

Let's imagine you have a report to read. When you're ready to read it, be very clear about your intention. Say to yourself: "I am reading this report now!" Then, start reading it.

Whenever you notice your mind wandering - whether to an external distraction or an internal thought or feeling – say to yourself, "Mind-wandering" or "Distraction." Then, return to reading the report. Distractions may occur anywhere from a few, to a dozen, to hundreds of times! Don't judge yourself: the brain naturally wanders. Each time it wanders, you have another chance to train it to focus. The more you do this, the better!

~ Elizabeth (Liz) Ahmann, ScD, RN, ACC.

Liz Ahmann, ScD, RN, ACC is an experienced ADHD Coach. She also teaches mindfulness classes for individuals with ADHD. Learn more at www.lizahmann.com www.lizahmann.com/mindfulness.html

Sticker Art Motivation Tip

Try this clever system to increase your motivation to complete "boring or unpleasant" tasks. Instead of using an electronic organizer, schedule the tasks in an agenda book or calendar. You may find others write down the to-do tasks, which improves memory and follow through.

Instead of just crossing the tasks off your to-do list, you can make completing the task more pleasurable by "rewarding" yourself when you finish. Buy some cute stickers in interesting shapes and colors. Reward yourself by placing a pretty sticker in your agenda or calendar when you complete the task.

You'll have a visual reminder of your success and create a work of art in the process! You can take it a step further and reward yourself with something special to pamper yourself when you earn enough stickers! Win-win!

~ Dr. Kari Miller, PhD, BCET

Dr. Kari Miller, ADHD coach and educational therapist, helps women focus and organize so they get more done and finish what they start! www.ADHDclearandfocused.com Kari.Miller.coach@gmail.com

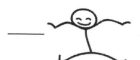

Extra Exploration Time

W hen our sons were little, the walk to school, less than a block away, could take half an hour. There were mud puddles, earthworms, leaves, plants and rocks on the ground— so much to see and do in everyday things. I picked the battle of allowing more exploration time and then giving them a 'count down' such as "two more rocks and then we have to go." That extra half hour in the morning meant getting up earlier (for me: they would be up and bouncing around early), getting things together and ready the night before and reminding myself to step back and try to see things through their eyes. The more I tried to hurry them up, the more slowly they would move. So...the less stressed I could appear, the more fun they would have, and the sooner they would get to school.

~ Pat Corbett, BEd, MC, MSW

Pat Corbett (mother and ally) hopes to help bridge the gaps and strengths for individuals and workers. Her new website is www.reframingthebox.com

Are You "Time Blind?"

"Where did the time go?" Lack of time awareness, not having a sense of time passing, or not being able to accurately estimate how long something will take to do are common challenges for people with ADHD. Most don't realize that their procrastination, overwhelm or inability to get things done is related to this "time blindness."

Being "time blind" is very real and can be understood by comparing it to people who are colorblind. People who are colorblind may never be able to differentiate between colors, but they learn strategies to compensate.

Being "time blind" is the same. Make sure your environment is full of time reminders. Go back to wearing a watch. Use alarms on your phone to go off every hour. Place analog clocks everywhere, including the bathroom, shower, garage and even your car.

~Laurie Dupar, PMHNP, RN, PCC

Laurie Dupar, PMHNP, RN, PCC is a trained Psychiatric Nurse Practitioner and 12 year veteran ADHD coach specializing in mentoring and training emerging ADHD Coaches.
www.coachingforadhd.com support@coachingforadhd.com

"Courage doesn't always roar, sometimes it's the quiet voice at the end of the day whispering, I will try again tomorrow."

~Mary Anne Radmacher

Want to be a <u>contributor</u> to the next edition of The ADHD Awareness Book Project?

- Do you have an ADHD success tip or strategy you want to share?

or

- Is there an ADHD story that you need to tell?

If so…

We would love to hear from you so you can be part of our next *Succeed with ADHD* book!

Go to:

www.CoachingforADHD.com

or email:

Support@CoachingforADHD.com

Made in the USA
San Bernardino, CA
11 October 2015